9.95

MANUAL OF EMERGENCY DRUGS

BRYAN E. BLEDSOE
Division of Emergency Medicine
Texas College of Osteopathic Medicine
North Texas State University
Fort Worth, Texas

Robert J. Brady Co., Bowie, Maryland 20715
A Prentice-Hall Publishing and Communications Company

Executive Editors: Richard A. Weimer/Jim Yvorra
Production Editor/Text Designer: Janis K. Oppelt
Art Director: Don Sellers, AMI
Typesetting: Creative Communications Corporation, Cockeysville, Maryland
Printed by: Kingsport Press, Kingsport, Tennessee

Manual of Emergency Drugs

For information, address Robert J. Brady Co., Bowie, Maryland 20715

Library of Congress Cataloging in Publication Data
Bledsoe, Bryan E., 1955-

Manual of emergency drugs.
Bibliography: p.
Includes index.
1. Medical emergencies—Handbooks, manuals, etc.
2. Drugs—Handbooks, manuals, etc. I. Title. [DNLM:
1. Emergencies—Handbooks. 2. Drug therapy—Handbooks.
WB330 B646m]
RC86.7.B595 1984 615.5'8 83-10034

ISBN 0-89303-647-1

Prentice-Hall International, Inc., London
Prentice-Hall Canada, Inc., Scarborough, Ontario
Prentice-Hall of Australia, Pty., Ltd., Sydney
Prentice-Hall of India Private Limited, New Delhi
Prentice-Hall of Japan, Inc., Tokyo
Prentice-Hall of Southeast Asia Pte. Ltd., Singapore
Whitehall Books, Limited, Petone, New Zealand
Editora Prentice-Hall Do Brasil LTDA., Rio de Janeiro

Printed in the United States of America

84 85 86 87 88 89 90 91 92 93 94 10 9 8 7 6 5 4 3 2 1

CONTENTS

PREFACE

Manual of Emergency Drugs was designed to provide emergency medical personnel with a handy reference to the most commonly used emergency medications. Chapter 1 profiles over 60 emergency medications in a standard, easy-to-read format. Chapter 2 lists the same medications by drug actions. The commonly used IV fluids, both crystalloids and colloids, are profiled in detail in Chapter 3. Chapter 4, Pediatric Emergency Drugs, contains a detailed breakdown of emergency medications by patient weight to help ensure correct and rapid drug administration when managing a pediatric emergency crisis. Chapter 5 provides a listing of over 1100 home medications, both prescription and nonprescription, to aid emergency personnel in elucidating patient drug histories. Overall, emergency medical personnel will find *Manual of Emergency Drugs* to be a useful and handy guide to many of the pharmacological agents encountered in prehospital and inhospital emergency care.

ACKNOWLEDGMENTS

A book, even the size of *Manual of Emergency Drugs*, requires the help and support of many dedicated persons. Special thanks goes to the publishing professionals at Brady including: Richard Weimer and Jim Yvorra, Executive Editors; Claire Merrick and Chuck Mondin, Sales and Marketing; and Janis Oppelt and Tony Melendez, Book Production. Special recognition must go to Janis who spent many hours looking up and correcting the many drug names presented in this text, correcting the grammar, and taking time to keep me up on the various stages of the manuscript.

There were many persons working with me at Texas College of Osteopathic Medicine who were always available to answer many of my never ending questions. Special thanks goes to Harbans Lal, Ph.D. and Edward Elko, Ph.D. National reviewers of this work included Kathleen Fitzgerald-Westby, R.N., Charles I. Craigmile, Gene C. Palmer, Ph.D., and Margaret Hardman, R.N., M.S.N. Gideon Bosker, M.D. of Portland, Oregon, and Frank J. Papa, D.O., of Fort Worth, Texas, proved invaluable in providing medical and technical assistance through all stages of production.

Thanks also go to Corky Baird of the Division of Evaluation Services at Texas College of Osteopathic Medicine for his assistance with the computer work used in the production of this manuscript.

Finally, special thanks to my wife Emma for her patience and help in typing and retyping the manuscript as well as her unending support.

This listing of prehospital drugs is derived from prehospital drug lists from across the United States. It does not constitute a recommendation by the author or the publisher of the drugs presented herein.

Although every attempt has been made to assure that the drug dosages and indications presented are in accordance with national standards and recommendations, neither the author or the publisher are responsible for any accidental deletions or discrepencies encountered.

1

QUICK DRUG REFERENCE

INTRODUCTION

This section provides a quick reference to over 60 of the most commonly used emergency medications. The dosages and indications have been taken from the most recent Advanced Cardiac Life Support (ACLS) standards of the American Heart Association. Drugs not covered in ACLS are taken from the American Medical Association's *Drug Evaluation*. It is important to keep in mind that specific drugs, dosages, indications, and routes may vary in your particular area. It is essential to be familiar with these variations and follow the guidelines established by the medical director of the system in which you work.

ACTIVATED CHARCOAL

class:	Adsorbent
actions:	Adsorbs toxins by chemical binding and large surface area
indications:	Poisoning following emesis or where emesis is contraindicated
contraindications:	None in severe poisoning
precautions:	Should only be administered following emesis in cases where it is so indicated
side effects:	Rare
dosage:	Two tablespoons (50 grams) mixed with a glass of water to form a slurry
route:	Oral
pediatric dosage:	Two tablespoons (50 grams) mixed with a glass of water to form a slurry

AMINOPHYLLINE

class:	Xanthine
actions:	Smooth muscle relaxant Causes bronchodilation Has mild diuretic properties Positive chronotrope
indications:	Bronchial asthma Reversible bronchospasm associated with chronic bronchitis and emphysema Congestive heart failure Pulmonary edema
contraindications:	Patients with history of hypersensitivity to the drug Hypotension Patients with peptic ulcer disease
precautions:	Monitor for arrhythmias Monitor blood pressure
side effects:	Convulsions Arrhythmias Vomiting Palpitations
dosage:	*METHOD 1.* 250-500 mg in 90 or 80 ml of D_5W respectively infused over 20-30 minutes

Aminophylline (continued)

METHOD 2. 250-500 mg (5-7 mg/kg) in 20 ml of D_5W infused over 20-30 minutes

route: Slow IV

pediatric dosage: *Status asthmaticus.* 3-4 mg/kg loading dose to be infused over 20-30 minutes. Maximum dose not to exceed 12 mg/kg per 24 hours.

AMYL NITRITE

class: Nitrate

actions: Causes coronary vasodilation
Removes cyanide-ion via complex mechanism

indications: Cyanide poisoning (bitter almond smell to breath)

contraindications: None when used in the management of cyanide poisoning

precautions: Hypotension
Has tendency for abuse

side effects: Headache
Nausea

dosage: Inhalant should be broken and inhaled, repeated as needed until patient is delivered to ED. Effects diminish after 20 minutes.

route: Inhalation

pediatric dosage: Inhalant should be broken and inhaled, repeated until patient is delivered to ED

ATROPINE

class:	Parasympatholytic
actions:	Blocks acetylcholine receptors Positive chronotrope Decreases GI secretions
indications:	Bradycardia Hypotension secondary to bradycardia Third degree heart block Asystole Organophosphate poisoning
contraindications:	None when used in emergency situations
precautions:	Dose of 2.0 mg should not be exceeded except in cases of organophosphate poisonings Tachycardia Hypertension
side effects:	Palpitations Headache Dry mouth
dosage:	*Bradycardia*. 0.5 mg every 5 minutes to a maximum of 2.0 mg *Asystole*. 1.0 mg *Organophosphate poisoning*. 2-5 mg

Atropine (continued)

route:	IV
pediatric dosage:	*Bradycardia*. 0.01-0.03 mg/kg *Organophosphate poisoning*. 0.05 mg/kg

BRETYLIUM (Bretylol®)

class:	Antiarrhythmic
actions:	Increases ventricular fibrillation threshold Blocks the release of norepinephrine from peripheral sympathetic nerves
indications:	Ventricular fibrillation refractory to lidocaine Ventricular tachycardia refractory to lidocaine
contraindications:	None when used in the management of life-threatening arrhythmias
precautions:	Postural hypotension occurs in approximately 50% of patients receiving Bretylium Patient must be kept supine Decrease dosage in patients being treated with catecholamine sympathomimetics
side effects:	Hypotension Increased frequency of arrhythmias

Bretylium (continued)

dosage:	5 mg/kg May be repeated at dose of 10 mg/kg up to a total dose of 30 mg/kg
route:	Rapid IV bolus
pediatric dosage:	Safety and efficacy in children has not been established

BUTOROPHANOL (Stadol®)

class:	Synthetic analgesic
actions:	CNS depressant Decreases sensitivity to pain 2 mg Stadol equivalent to 10 mg morphine
indications:	Moderate to severe pain
contraindications:	Patients with a history of hypersensitivity to the drug Head injury Use with caution in patients with impaired respiratory function
precautions:	Respiratory depression (Narcan® should be available) Patients dependent on narcotics
side effects:	May experience symptoms of withdrawal Nausea Dizziness Altered levels of consciousness
dosage:	*IV.* 1 mg *IM.* 2 mg
routes:	IV IM
pediatric dosage:	Rarely used

CALCIUM CHLORIDE

class:	Electrolyte
actions:	Positive inotrope Increases myocardial automaticity
indications:	Asystole Electromechanical dissociation Abdominal muscle spasm associated with spider bite and Man-O-War stings
contraindications:	Patients receiving digitalis
precautions:	IV line should be flushed between calcium chloride and sodium bicarbonate
side effects:	Few
dosage:	250-500 mg (2.5-5.0 ml of 10% solution)
routes:	IV IC
pediatric dosage:	20 mg/kg

CHLORPROMAZINE (Thorazine®)

class:	Major tranquilizer
actions:	Blocks dopamine receptors in brain associated with mood and behavior Has antiemetic properties
indications:	Acute psychotic episodes Mild alcohol withdrawal Intractible hiccoughs Nausea and vomiting
contraindications:	Comatose states Should not be administered in the presence of sedatives Should not be administered in the presence of hallucinogens or phenycyclidine-like compounds
precautions:	Orthostatic hypotension May cause extrapyramidal reactions (Parkinson-like), especially in children
side effects:	Physical and mental impairment Drowsiness
dosage:	25 mg
route:	IM
pediatric dosage:	0.5 mg/kg

DESLANOSIDE (Cedilanid-D®)

class: Cardiac Glycoside

actions: Positive inotrope
Increases cardiac output
Reduces edema associated with CHF

indications: Acute congestive heart failure
Rapid atrial arrhythmias, especially atrial flutter and atrial fibrillation, that cause hemodynamic compromise

contraindications: Any patients with signs or symptoms of digitalis toxicity
Ventricular fibrillation

precautions: Monitor for signs of digitalis toxicity
Patients who have recently suffered an MI have greater sensitivity to the effects of digitalis
Calcium should not be administered to patients on digitalis

side effects: Nausea
Vomiting

dosage: 0.8-1.6 mg

routes: IM
IV slowly

pediatric dosage: 0.025 mg/kg

DEXAMETHASONE (Decadron®)

class:	Steroid
actions:	Decreases cerebral edema Anti-inflammatory Suppresses immune response (especially in allergic/anaphylactic reactions)
indications:	Cerebral edema Possibly effective as an adjunctive agent in the management of shock
contraindications:	None in the emergency setting
precautions:	Should be protected from heat Onset of action may be 2-6 hours and thus should not be considered to be of use in the critical first hour following an anaphylactic reaction.
side effects:	GI bleeding Prolonged wound healing
dosage:	4-24 mg
route:	IV
pediatric dosage:	1 mg/kg

50% DEXTROSE

class:	Carbohydrate
actions:	Elevates blood glucose level rapidly
indications:	Hypoglycemia Coma of unknown origin
contraindications:	None in the emergency setting
precautions:	Dextrostix must be performed and blood sample drawn before administration
side effects:	Local venous irritation
dosage:	25 grams (50 ml)
route:	IV
pediatric dosage:	0.5-1 gm/kg slow IV

DIAZEPAM (Valium®)

class:	Tranquilizer
actions:	Anticonvulsant Skeletal muscle relaxant Sedative
indications:	Major motor seizures Status epilepticus Premedication prior to cardioversion Skeletal muscle relaxant Acute anxiety states
contraindications:	Patients with a history of hypersensitivity to the drug
precautions:	Can cause local venous irritation Has short duration of effect Do not mix with other drugs due to possible precipitation problems
side effects:	Drowsiness Hypotension Respiratory depression
dosage:	*Status epilepticus.* 5-10 mg IV *Acute anxiety.* 2-5 mg IM or IV *Premedication prior to cardioversion.* 5-15 mg IV

Diazepam (continued)

routes:

IV (care must be taken not to administer faster than 1 milliliter/minute)
IM

pediatric dosage:

Status epilepticus. 0.5-2.0 mg

DIAZOXIDE (Hyperstat®)

class:	Antihypertensive
actions:	Causes decrease in both systolic and diastolic pressure Direct peripheral arteriole dilation
indications:	Malignant hypertensive crisis
contraindications:	None in the emergency setting
precautions:	Avoid overcorrection of blood pressure Blood pressure must be constantly monitored Patient should be supine
side effects:	Hypotension Syncope Local venous irritation
dosage:	300 mg IV within 30 seconds
route:	IV only
pediatric dosage:	5 mg/kg

DIGOXIN (Lanoxin®)

class:	Cardiac Glycoside
actions:	Positive inotrope Increases cardiac output Reduces edema associated with CHF
indications:	CHF Rapid atrial arrhythmias, especially atrial flutter and atrial fibrillation
contraindications:	Any patient with signs or symptoms of digitalis toxicity Ventricular fibrillation
precautions:	Monitor for signs of digitalis toxicity Patients who have recently suffered an MI have greater sensitivity to the effects of digitalis Calcium should not be administered to patients receiving digitalis
side effects:	Nausea Vomiting
dosage:	0.25-0.50 mg
route:	IV
pediatric dosage:	25-40 mcg/kg

DIPHENHYDRAMINE (Benadryl®)

class:	Antihistamine
actions:	Blocks histamine receptors Has some sedative effects
indications:	Anaphylaxis Allergic reactions
contraindications:	Asthma Nursing mothers
precautions:	Hypotension
side effects:	Sedation Drys bronchial secretions Blurred vision Headache Palpitations
dosage:	25-50 mg
routes:	Slow IV push Deep IM
pediatric dosage:	2-5 mg/kg

DOBUTAMINE (Dobutrex®)

class:	Sympathomimetic
actions:	Positive inotrope Little chronotropic activity
indications:	Short-term management of CHF
contraindications:	Should only be used in patients with an adequate heart rate
precautions:	Ventricular irritability Use with caution following MI Can be deactivated by alkaline solutions
side effects:	Increased heart rate Palpitations
dosage:	2.5-10 micrograms/kg/minute *METHOD.* 250 milligrams should be placed in 500 milliliters of D_5W. This gives a concentration of 0.5 mg/ml.
route:	IV drip
pediatric dosage:	Rarely used

DOPAMINE (Intropin®)
(See Dosage Chart on page 24-25)

class:	Sympathomimetic
actions:	Positive inotrope Selectively dilates blood vessels of kidney, mesentery, brain, and heart
indications:	Cardiogenic shock Hypovolemic shock (only after complete fluid resuscitation)
contraindications:	Hypovolemic shock where complete fluid resuscitation has not occurred
precautions:	Should not be administered in the presence of severe tachyarrhythmias Should not be administered in the presence of ventricular fibrillation Ventricular irritability
side effects:	Ventricular tachyarrhythmias Hypertension
dosage:	5-20 micrograms/kg/minute *METHOD.* 800 milligrams should be placed in 500 ml of D_5W giving a concentration of 1600 micrograms/ml
route:	IV drip only
pediatric dosage	2-10 mcg/kg/minute

TABLE 1-1. INTROPIN® (DOPAMI

FOR A CONCENTRATION OF 1600 mcg DOPAMINE H

BODY WT lbs	77	88	99	110	121	132	1
kgs	35	40	45	50	55	60	6
FLOW RATE IN DROPS* PER MINUTE							
5	3.8	3.4	2.9	2.6	2.4	2.2	2
10	7.6	6.7	5.9	5.3	4.9	4.5	4
15	11	10	8.9	8.0	7.3	6.6	6
20	15	13	12	11	9.7	8.9	8
25	19	17	15	13	12	11	1
30	23	20	18	16	15	13	1
35	27	23	21	19	17	16	1
40	31	27	24	21	19	18	1
45	34	30	27	24	22	20	1
50	38	33	30	27	24	22	2
55	42	37	33	29	27	24	2
60	46	40	36	32	29	27	2
70	53	47	42	37	34	31	2
80	61	53	47	43	39	36	3
90	69	60	53	48	44	40	3
100	76	67	59	53	49	45	4

DOSAGE = m

*Based on a microdrip calibration of 60 drops equal to 1.0 milliliter

Note: All dosages of 10 mcg/kg/min and above have been rounded off to the near mcg/kg/min.

(Courtesy of American Critical Care, Division of American Hospital Supply Corpo tion, McGaw Park, Illinois)

Cl) DOSAGE CHART

) mg INTROPIN PER 500 ml—OR—400 mg INTROPIN PER 250 ml)

54	165	176	187	198	209	220	231	242
70	75	80	85	90	95	100	105	110
.9	1.8	1.6	1.55	1.5	1.4	1.3	1.25	1.2
.8	3.6	3.3	3.1	3.0	2.8	2.7	2.5	2.4
.7	5.3	5.0	4.7	4.4	4.2	4.0	3.8	3.6
.6	7.1	6.7	6.3	5.9	5.6	5.3	5.1	4.9
.5	8.9	8.4	7.8	7.4	7.0	6.6	6.3	6.0
11	11	10	9.4	8.9	8.4	8.0	7.6	7.3
13	12	12	11	10	9.8	9.3	8.9	8.5
15	14	13	13	12	11	11	10	9.7
17	16	15	14	13	13	12	11	11
19	18	17	16	15	14	13	13	12
21	20	18	17	16	15	15	14	13
23	21	20	19	18	17	16	15	15
27	25	23	22	21	20	19	18	17
31	28	27	25	24	23	21	20	19
34	32	30	28	27	25	24	23	22
38	36	33	31	30	28	27	25	24

OPAMINE HCl/kg/min

EDROPHONIUM (Tensilon®)

class:	Anticholinesterase
actions:	Inhibits action of enzyme cholinesterase thus potentiating acetylcholine Increases parasympathetic tone
indications:	PSVT refractory to vagal maneuvers
contraindications:	Patients with a history of hypersensitivity to the drug
precautions:	Respiratory pattern must be constantly monitored Bradycardia Hypotension Avoid exposure to dextrose solutions
side effects:	Dizziness Syncope
dosage:	5 mg IV
route:	IV
pediatric dosage:	2 mg IV followed by carotid massage

EPINEPHRINE 1:1000

class:	Sympathomimetic
actions:	Bronchodilation Positive chronotrope Positive inotrope
indications:	Bronchial asthma Exacerbation of some forms of chronic obstructive pulmonary disease (COPD) Anaphylaxis
contraindications:	Patients with underlying cardiovascular disease Hypertension Pregnancy Patients with tachyarrhythmias
precautions:	Should be protected from light Blood pressure, pulse, and EKG must be constantly monitored
side effects:	Palpitations Anxiousness Headache
dosage:	0.3-0.5 mg
route:	Subcutaneously
pediatric dosage:	0.01 mg/kg up to 0.3 mg

EPINEPHRINE 1:10,000

class: Sympathomimetic

actions: Positive chronotrope
Positive inotrope
Causes bronchodilation

indications: Fine ventricular fibrillation
Asystole
Electromechanical dissociation

contraindications: None when used in the situations listed above

precautions: Should be protected from light
Can be deactivated by alkaline solutions

side effects: Tachyarrhythmias

dosages: *Cardiac Arrest.* 0.5 mg (5 ml) repeated every five minutes
Severe anaphylaxis. 0.3-0.5 mg (3-5 ml)

routes: IV
Transtracheal
Intracardiac (not recommended)

pediatric dosage: 0.01 mg/kg repeated every five minutes

EPINEPHRINE SUSPENSION (Sus-Phrine®)

class:	Sympathomimetic
actions:	Bronchodilation Positive chronotrope Positive inotrope
indications:	Bronchial Asthma Anaphylaxis
contraindications:	Patients with underlying cardiovascular disease Pregnancy Patients with tachyarrhythmias
precautions:	Should be protected from light Blood pressure, pulse, and EKG must be constantly monitored
side effects:	Palpitations Anxiousness Headache
dosage:	0.1-0.3
route:	Subcutaneously
pediatric dosage:	0.005 ml/kg

RACEMIC EPINEPHRINE (microNEFRIN®)

class:	Sympathomimetic
actions:	Bronchodilation Positive chronotrope Positive inotrope
indications:	Croup (laryngotracheobronchitis)
contraindications:	Epiglottitis Hypersensitivity to the drug
precautions:	Vital signs should be constantly monitored Should be used only once
side effects:	Palpitations Anxiety Headache
dosage:	5-6 inhalations
route:	Inhalation only
pediatric dosage:	5-6 inhalations

ETHACRYNIC ACID (Edecrin®)

class:	Potent diuretic
actions:	Inhibits readsorption of sodium chloride Promotes prompt diuresis Vasodilation
indications:	Congestive heart failure Pulmonary edema
contraindications:	Pregnancy Dehydration
precautions:	Should be protected from light Dehydration
side effects:	Transient deafness
dosage:	50 mg (drug must be reconstituted before use)
route:	IV
pediatric dosage:	Not indicated

FUROSEMIDE (Lasix®)

class:	Potent diuretic
actions:	Inhibits readsorption of sodium chloride Promotes prompt diuresis Vasodilation
indications:	Congestive heart failure Pulmonary edema
contraindications:	Pregnancy Dehydration
precautions:	Should be protected from light Dehydration
side effects:	Few in emergency usage
dosage:	40-80 mg
route:	IV
pediatric dosage:	1 mg/kg

GLUCAGON

class:	Antihypoglycemic agent
actions:	Causes breakdown of glycogen to glucose Inhibits glycogen synthesis Elevates blood glucose level Positive inotrope Positive chronotrope
indications:	Hypoglycemia
contraindications:	Hypersensitivity to the drug
precautions:	Only effective if there are sufficient stores of glycogen within the liver Use with caution in patients with cardiovascular or renal disease Draw blood glucose prior to administration
side effects:	Few in emergency situations
dosage:	O.5-1.0 units
routes:	IV IM
pediatric dosage:	Rarely used

GLUCOLA

class:	Carbohydrate
actions:	Increases blood glucose level
indications:	Conscious patients with suspected hypoglycemia
contraindications:	Any patient who is not conscious enough to drink without assistance
precautions:	Monitor airway Draw blood glucose prior to administration
side effects:	Nausea Vomiting
dosage:	Sipped until patient feels improvement (50-200 ml)
route:	Oral
pediatric dosage:	Sipped until patient feels improvement

HALOPERIDOL (Haldol®)

class:	Major tranquilizer
actions:	Blocks dopamine receptors in brain responsible for mood and behavior Has antiemetic properties
indications:	Acute psychotic episodes
contraindications:	Should not be administered in the presence of other sedatives Should not be used in the management of dysphoria caused by Talwin®
precautions:	Orthostatic hypotension
side effects:	Physical and mental impairment Parkinson-like reactions have been known to occur, especially in children
dosage:	2-5 mg
route:	IM
pediatric dosage:	Rarely used

HYDROCORTISONE (Solu-Cortef®)

class:	Steroid
actions:	Anti-inflammatory Suppresses immune response (especially in allergic/ anaphylactic reactions)
indications:	Severe anaphylaxis Possibly effective as an adjunctive agent in the management of shock
contraindications:	None in the emergency setting
precautions:	Must be reconstituted and used promptly Onset of action may be 2-6 hours and thus should not be expected to be of use in the critical first hour following an acute anaphylactic reaction.
side effects:	GI bleeding Prolonged wound healing Suppression of natural steroids
dosage:	100-250 mg
routes:	IM IV
pediatric dosage:	30 mcg/kg

HYDROMORPHONE (Dilaudid®)

class: Narcotic

actions:
- CNS depressant
- Causes some peripheral vasodilation
- Decreases sensitivity to pain

indications:
- Severe pain
- Pulmonary edema

contraindications:
- Head injury
- Volume depletion
- Undiagnosed abdominal pain
- Patients with history of hypersensitivity to the drug

precautions:
- Respiratory depression (Narcan® should be available)
- Hypotension
- Nausea

side effects:
- Dizziness
- Altered level of consciousness

dosage: 1 mg

routes:
- IV
- IM

pediatric dosage: Rarely used

HYDROXYZINE (Vistaril®)

class:	Antihistamine
actions:	Antiemetic Antihistamine Antianxiety Potentiates analgesic effects of narcotics and related agents
indications:	To potentiate the effects of narcotics and synthetic narcotics Nausea and vomiting Anxiety reactions
contraindications:	Patients with a history of hypersensitivity to the drug
precautions:	Orthostatic hypotension Analgesic dosages should be reduced when used with Vistaril®
side effects:	Drowsiness
dosage:	50-100 mg
route:	Deep IM only
pediatric dosage:	1 mg/kg

INSULIN

class:	Hypoglycemic agent
actions:	Causes uptake of glucose by the cells Decreases blood glucose level Promotes glucose storage
indications:	Diabetic ketoacidosis
contraindications:	Avoid overcompensation of blood glucose level If possible, administration should wait until the patient is in the emergency department
precautions:	Administration of excessive dose may induce hypoglycemia. Glucose should be available.
side effects:	Few in emergency situations
dosage:	10-25 units regular insulin IV followed by an infusion at 0.1 units/kg/hour
route:	IV
pediatric dosage:	Dosage is based on each individual case

IPECAC

class:	Emetic
actions:	Irritates the enteric tract Stimulates vomiting center
indications:	Poisoning in conscious patient
contraindications:	Vomiting should not be induced in any patient with impaired consciousness Poisonings involving strong acids, bases, or petroleum distillates Antiemetic poisonings, especially of the phenothiazine type
precautions:	Monitor and assure a patent airway
side effects:	Rare
dosage:	30 ml (1 ounce) followed by several glasses of warm water
route:	Oral
pediatric dosage:	*Less than 1 year of age.* 5-10 ml *Greater than 1 year of age.* 15 ml repeated in 20 minutes

ISOETHARINE (Bronkosol®)

class:	Sympathomimetic
actions:	Bronchodilation Some positive chronotropic properties
indications:	Bronchial asthma Reversible bronchospasm associated with chronic bronchitis and emphysema
contraindications:	Patients with history of hypersensitivity to the drug
precautions:	Blood pressure, pulse, and EKG must be constantly monitored
side effects:	Palpitations Anxiousness Headache
dosage:	*Hand nebulizer*. 4 inhalations *Oxygen aerosolization*. 0.5 ml (1:3 with saline) *IPPB*. 0.5 ml (1:3 with saline)
route:	Inhalation only
pediatric dosage:	Rarely used

ISOPROTERENOL (Isuprel®)

class: Sympathomimetic

actions:
Positive chronotrope
Positive inotrope
Causes bronchodilation

indications:
Bradycardias refractory to atropine
Bradycardias due to high-degree heart blocks
Asystole

contraindications: Should not be used to increase blood pressure in cardiogenic shock

precautions:
Can cause ventricular irritability
Can be deactivated by alkaline solutions
Should be used with caution in recent MI

side effects:
Tachyarrhythmias
Palpitations

dosage: 1 mg should be placed in 500 ml of D_5W. This should then be slowly infused and titrated until the desired rate is obtained or until PVCs occur.

route: IV drip only

pediatric dosage: 0.1 mcg/kg/minute

LIDOCAINE (Xylocaine®)

class:	Antiarrhythmic
actions:	Suppresses ventricular ectopic activity Increases ventricular fibrillation threshold Reduces velocity of electrical impulse through conductive system
indications:	Malignant PVCs Ventricular tachycardia Ventricular fibrillation
contraindications:	High degree heart blocks PVCs in conjunction with bradycardia
precautions:	Dosage should not exceed 300 mg/hr Monitor for CNS toxicity Bolus should be followed by an infusion
side effects:	Anxiety Nausea Convulsions Widening of QRS

Lidocaine (continued)

dosage:	*BOLUS.* Initial bolus of 50-75 mg followed by two subsequent boluses of 50-75 mg every 10 minutes to achieve a maximum loading dose of 225 mg over 20 minutes *DRIP.* 2-4 mg/minute
routes:	IV Push IV Drip
pediatric dosage:	1 mg/kg

MAGNESIUM SULFATE

class:	Anticonvulsant
actions:	CNS depressant Anticonvulsant
indications:	Seizures accompanying eclampsia (toxemia of pregnancy)
contraindications:	Any patient with heart block or recent MI
precautions:	Caution should be used in patients receiving digitalis Hypotension Calcium chloride should be readily available as an antidote if respiratory depression ensues
side effects:	Respiratory depression Drowsiness
dosage:	1-4 gms
route:	IV
pediatric dosage:	Not indicated

MANNITOL (Osmitrol®)

class:	Osmotic diuretic
actions:	Draws fluid from intracellular space into extracellular space Increases urinary output
indications:	Acute cerebral edema Blood transfusion reactions
contraindications:	Pulmonary edema Patients who are dehydrated Hypersensitivity to the drug
precautions:	Rapid administration can cause circulatory overload Crystallization of the drug can occur at lower temperatures An in-line filter should be used
side effects:	Pulmonary congestion Sodium depletion
dosage:	500 ml of a 20% solution administered over 30-60 minutes
route:	IV drip
pediatric dosage:	250 mg/kg IV over 5 minutes

MEPERIDINE (Demerol®)

class:	Narcotic
actions:	CNS depressant Decreases sensitivity to pain
indications:	Severe pain
contraindications:	Patients receiving monoamine oxidase inhibitors Undiagnosed abdominal pain Patients with history of hypersensitivity to the drug
precautions:	Respiratory depression (Narcan® should be available) Hypotension Nausea
side effects:	Dizziness Altered level of consciousness
dosage:	*IV.* 25-50 mg *IM.* 50-100 mg
routes:	IV IM
pediatric dosage:	1 mg/kg

METARAMINOL (Aramine®)

class:	Sympathomimetic
actions:	Causes release of endogenous stores of norepinephrine Positive inotrope
indications:	Cardiogenic shock
contraindications:	Hypotensive states due to hypovolemia
precautions:	Constant monitoring of blood pressure is essential Not effective in catecholamine depleted patients
side effects:	Palpitations Hypertension
dosage:	200 mg should be placed in 500 ml of D_5W. This gives a concentration of 0.4 mg/ml which should be slowly infused and titrated to blood pressure response.
route:	IV drip only
pediatric dosages:	0.4 mg/kg/minute

METHYLPREDNISOLONE (Solu-Medrol®)

class:	Steroid
actions:	Anti-inflammatory Suppresses immune response (especially in allergic/anaphylactic reactions)
indications:	Severe anaphylaxis Possibly effective as an adjunctive agent in the management of shock
contraindications:	None in the emergency setting
precautions:	Must be reconstituted and used promptly Onset of action may be 2-6 hours and thus should not be expected to be of use in the critical first hour following an anaphylactic reaction.
side effects:	GI bleeding Prolonged wound healing Suppression of natural steroids
dosage:	125-250 mg
routes:	IV IM
pediatric dosage:	30 mcg/kg

MORPHINE

class:	Narcotic
actions:	CNS depressant Causes peripheral vasodilation Decreases sensitivity to pain
indications:	Severe pain Pulmonary edema
contraindications:	Head injury Volume depletion Undiagnosed abdominal pain Patients with history of hypersensitivity to the drug
precautions:	Respiratory depression (Narcan® should be available) Hypotension Nausea
side effects:	Dizziness Altered level of consciousness
dosage:	*IV.* 2-5 mg followed by 2 mg every few minutes until the pain is relieved or until respiratory depression ensues *IM.* 5-15 mg based on patient weight
routes:	IV IM
pediatric dosage:	0.1-0.2 mg/kg IV

NALBUPHINE (Nubain®)

class:	Synthetic analgesic
actions:	CNS depressant Decreases sensitivity to pain
indications:	Moderate to severe pain
contraindications:	Patients with a history of hypersensitivity to the drug
precautions:	Use with caution in patients with impaired respiratory function Respiratory depression (Narcan® should be available) Patients dependent on narcotics May experience symptoms of withdrawal Nausea
side effects:	Dizziness Altered level of consciousness
dosage:	5-10 mg
routes:	IV IM
pediatric dosage:	Rarely used

NALOXONE (Narcan®)

class: Narcotic antagonist

actions: Reverses effects of narcotics

indications: Narcotic overdoses including:

morphine	Paregoric
Dilaudid®	methadone
fentanyl	heroin
Demerol®	Percodan®

Synthetic analgesic overdoses including:

Nubain®	Talwin®
Stadol®	Darvon®

Alcoholic coma

To rule out narcotics in coma of unknown origin

contraindications: Patients with a history of hypersensitivity to the drug

precautions: Should be administered with caution to patients dependent on narcotics as it may cause withdrawal effects

Short-acting, should be augmented every 5 minutes

side effects: None

dosage: 0.4-2.0 mg up to a total dose of 10 mg (larger doses may be required to reverse effects of Darvon®)

Naloxone (continued)

routes: IV
IM

pediatric dosage: 0.005 mg/kg

NITROGLYCERIN (Nitrostat®)

class:	Antianginal
actions:	Dilates coronary arteries Dilates systemic arteries
indications:	Angina pectoris Chest pain associated with MI
contraindications:	Children under 12 Hypotension
precautions:	Constantly monitor blood pressure Syncope Drug must be protected from light Expires quickly once bottle is opened
side effects:	Headache Dizziness Hypotension
dosage:	1 tablet repeated up to three times
route:	Sublingual
pediatric dosage:	Not indicated

NITROPASTE (Nitro-Bid®)

class:	Antianginal
actions:	Dilates coronary arteries Dilates systemic arteries
indications:	Angina pectoris Chest pain associated with MI
contraindications:	Children under 12 Hypotension
precautions:	Constantly monitor blood pressure Syncope Drug must be protected from light Expires quickly once bottle is opened
side effects:	Dizziness Hypotension
dosage:	1/2 to 3/4 inches
route:	Topical
pediatric dosage:	Not indicated

NITROUS-OXIDE (Nitronox®)

class:	Anesthetic gas
actions:	CNS depressant Decreases sensitivity to pain
indications:	Moderate to severe pain
contraindications:	Severe head injury
precautions:	Should be self-administered
side effects:	Nausea Vomiting Bizarre behavior
dosage:	Self-administered
route:	Inhalation (50% oxygen/50% nitrous-oxide mixture)
pediatric dosage:	Self-administered

NOREPINEPHRINE (Levophed®)

class:	Sympathomimetic
actions:	Causes peripheral vasoconstriction
indications:	Cardiogenic shock Neurogenic shock
contraindications:	Hypotensive states due to hypovolemia
precautions:	Can be deactivated by alkaline solutions Constant monitoring of blood pressure is essential
side effects:	Palpitations Hypertension Local venous irritation
dosage:	32-48 mcg/minute *METHOD.* 8 mg should be placed in 500 ml of D_5W giving a concentration of 16 mcg/ml. 2-3 ml should be delivered per minute.
route:	IV drip only
pediatric dosage:	2-4 mg should be placed in 500 ml of D_5W. This should be titrated to blood pressure response.

OXYTOCIN (Pitocin®)

class:	Oxytocic
actions:	Causes uterine contraction Causes lactation Slows post-partum vaginal bleeding
indications:	Post-partum vaginal bleeding
contraindications:	Any condition other than post-partum bleeding Cesarean section
precautions:	It is essential to assure that the placenta has delivered and that there is not another fetus present before administering oxytocin Overdosage can cause uterine rupture Hypertension
side effects:	Anaphylaxis Cardiac arrhythmias
dosage:	*IM.* 3-10 units *IV.* 10-20 units in 500 ml of D_5W administered according to uterine response
routes:	IM IV drip
pediatric dosage:	Not indicated

PENTAZOCINE (Talwin®)

class:	Synthetic Analgesic
actions:	CNS depressant Decreases sensitivity to pain
indications:	Moderate to severe pain
contraindications:	Patients with a history of hypersensitivity to the drug
precautions:	Use with caution in patients with impaired respiratory function Respiratory depression (Narcan® should be available) Patients dependent on narcotics May experience symptoms of withdrawal
side effects:	Nausea Dizziness Altered level of consciousness Hallucinations
dosage:	30 mg
routes:	IV IM
pediatric dosage:	Rarely used

PHENOBARBITAL

class:	Barbiturate
actions:	Suppresses spread of seizure activity through the motor cortex CNS depressant
indications:	Major motor seizures Status epilepticus Acute anxiety states
contraindications:	History of hypersensitivity to the drug
precautions:	Respiratory depression Hypotension Can cause hyperactivity in children
side effects:	Drowsiness Children may become hyperactive
dosage:	100-250 mg
route:	IV
pediatric dosage:	3-5 mg/kg

PHENYTOIN (Dilantin®)

class:	Anticonvulsant
actions:	Inhibits spread of seizure activity through motor cortex
indications:	Major motor seizures Status epilepticus Arrhythmias due to digitalis toxicity
contraindications:	Any arrhythmia except those due to digitalis toxicity Patients with history of hypersensitivity to the drug
precautions:	Should not be administered with sugar solutions Hypotension
side effects:	Local venous irritation CNS depression
dosage:	*Status epilepticus.* 150-250 mg (10-15 mg/kg) not to exceed 25 mg/minute *Digitalis toxicity.* 100 mg over 5 minutes can be repeated up to 1 gram until the arrhythmia is suppressed or until symptoms of CNS depression occur

route: IV

pediatric dosage: *Status epilepticus.* 8-10 mg/kg IV
Digitalis toxicity. 3-5 mg/kg IV over 5 minutes to a maximum dose of 50 mg

PHYSOSTIGMINE (Antilirium®)

class:	Cholinesterase inhibitor
actions:	Inhibits cholinsterase Potentiates acetylcholine
indications:	Tricyclic overdoses including: Tofranil® Norpramin® Elavil® Adapin® Sinequan® Atropine/Belladona overdoses
contraindications:	Asthma and COPD Gangrene Diabetics Cardiovascular disease
precautions:	Monitor for bronchospasm and laryngospasm Seizures
side effects:	Excessive salivation Bradycardia Emesis
dosage:	0.5-2.0 mg
route:	IV
pediatric dosage:	0.5-1.0 mg over 5 minutes

PRALIDOXIME (2-PAM) (Protopam®)

class:	Cholinesterase reactivator
actions:	Reactivates cholinesterase in cases of organophosphate poisoning Allows deactivation of accumulated acetylcholine Detoxifies certain organophosphates by direct chemical reaction
indications:	Severe organophosphate poisoning as characterized by muscle twitching, respiratory depression, and paralysis
contraindications:	Poisonings due to inorganic phosphates Poisonings other than organophosphates
precautions:	Laryngospasm, tachycardia and muscle rigidity have occurred following rapid administration Should only follow atropinization
side effects:	Excitement Manic behavior
dosage:	1 gm in 250-500 ml of normal saline infused over 30 minutes

route: IV drip

pediatric dosage: 20-40 mg/kg by the same mechanism

PROCAINAMIDE (Pronestyl®)

class:	Antiarrhythmic
actions:	Slows conduction through myocardium Elevates ventricular fibrillation threshold Suppresses ventricular ectopic activity
indications:	PVCs refractory to lidocaine Ventricular tachycardia refractory to lidocaine
contraindications:	High-degree heart blocks PVCs in conjunction with bradycardia
precautions:	Dosage should not exceed 1 gm Monitor for CNS toxicity
side effects:	Anxiety Nausea Convulsions Widening of QRS
dosage:	*INITIAL.* 20 mg/minute until: 1) Arrhythmia abolished 2) Hypotension ensues 3) QRS widened by 50% of original width 4) Total of 1 gm has been given *MAINTENANCE.* 1-4 mg/minute

Procainamide (continued)

routes:	Slow IV bolus IV drip
pediatric dosage:	Rarely used

PROMETHAZINE (Phenergan®)

class:	Antihistamine (H_1 antagonist)
actions:	Mild anticholinergic activity Antiemetic Potentiates actions of analgesics
indications:	Nausea and vomiting Motion sickness To potentiate the effects of analgesics
contraindications:	Comatose states Patients who have received a large amount of depressants
precautions:	Avoid accidental intra-arterial injection
side effects:	May impair mental and physical ability Drowsiness
dosage:	25 mg
route:	IV
pediatric dosage:	0.5 mg/kg

PROPRANOLOL (Inderal®)

class: Sympathetic blocker

action: Non-selectively blocks beta adrenergic receptors

indications:
Ventricular tachyarrhythmias refractory to lidocaine
Ventricular fibrillation refractory to lidocaine
Tachyarrhythmias due to digitalis toxicity

contraindications:
Asthmatics
Patients dependent on sympathetic agonists

precautions:
Should not be given concurrently with verapamil
Atropine and isoproterenol should be readily available

side effects:
Bradycardia
Heart blocks
CHF
Bronchospasm

dosages: 1-3 mg diluted in 10-30 ml of D_5W given slowly IV

route: Slow IV bolus

pediatric dosage: 0.01 mg/kg

SODIUM BICARBONATE

class:	Alkalinizing agent
actions:	Combines with excessive acids to form a weak volatile acid Increase pH
indications:	Severe acidosis Cardiac arrest Tricyclic antidepressant overdose
contraindications:	Alkalotic states
precautions:	Correct dosage is essential to avoid overcompensation of pH Can deactivate catecholamines Can precipitate with calcium
side effects:	Alkalosis
dosage:	1 mEq/kg initially followed by 1/2 mEq/kg every 10 minutes until blood gas studies are available
route:	IV
pediatric dosage:	1 mEq/kg initially followed by 1/2 mEq/kg every 10 minutes

SUCCINYLCHOLINE (Anectine®)

class:	Neuromuscular blocking agent
actions:	Skeletal muscle relaxant Motor nerve depolarization
indications:	Temporary paralysis where ET intubation is indicated and where muscle tone prevents it
contraindications:	Patients with a history of hypersensitivity to the drug
precautions:	Do not administer unless personnel skilled in ET intubation are present Endotracheal intubation equipment must be available Oxygen equipment and emergency resuscitative drugs must be available Paralysis occurs within one minute and lasts for approximately eight minutes
side effects:	Prolonged paralysis Hypotension Bradycardia
dosage:	1 mg/kg (20-80 mg in the adult)

Succinylcholine (continued)

route:	IV IM
pediatric dosage:	1 mg/kg

TERBUTALINE (Brethine®)

class:	Sympathomimetic
actions:	Bronchodilation Minor chronotropic properties
indications:	Bronchial asthma Reversible bronchospasm associated with chronic bronchitis and emphysema
contraindications:	Patients with history of hypersensitivity to the drug
precautions:	Blood pressure, pulse, and EKG must be constantly monitored
side effects:	Palpitations Anxiousness Headache
dosage:	0.25 mg
route:	Subcutaneous
pediatric dosage:	Not recommended

THIAMINE (Vitamin B1)

class:	Vitamin
actions:	Allows normal breakdown of glucose
indications:	Coma of unknown origin (especially if alcohol or malnourishment may be involved) Delirium tremens
contraindications:	None
precautions:	Occasional anaphylactic reactions have been reported
side effects:	Rare, if any
dosage:	100 mg
route:	IV
pediatric dosage:	Rarely used

VERAPAMIL (Isoptin®)

class:	Calcium-ion antagonist
actions:	Slows conduction through the AV node Inhibits reentry during PSVT Decreases the rate of the ventricular response Decreases myocardial oxygen demand Dilates coronary and peripheral arteries
indications:	PSVT Atrial flutter with rapid ventricular response Atrial fibrillation with rapid ventricular response
contraindications:	Heart block Conduction system disturbances
precautions:	Should not be used in patients receiving propranolol Hypotension
side effects:	Nausea Vomiting
dosage:	0.075-0.15 mg/kg (maximum of 10 mg)

route: IV

pediatric dosage:

0-1 year: 0.1-0.2 mg/kg (maximum of 2.0 mg) administered over one minute

1-15 years. 0.1-0.3 mg/kg (maximum of 5.0 mg) administered over one minute

2

EMERGENCY DRUGS BY CLASSIFICATION

CLASSIFICATION

positive chronotropic:	aminophylline atropine sulfate calcium chloride dobutamine dopamine epinephrine glucagon isoetharine isoproterenol metaraminol norepinephrine terbutaline
positive inotropic:	aminophylline calcium chloride digitalis dobutamine dopamine epinephrine glucagon isoetharine isoproterenol metaraminol norepinephrine terbutaline
negative chronotropic:	bretylium edrophonium lidocaine phenytoin procainamide verapamil

negative inotropic:	lidocaine procainamide propranolol
narcotics:	hydromorphone meperidine morphine
sedative/hypnotics:	chlorpromazine diazepam haloperidol phenytoin phenobarbital
antihistamines:	diphenhydramine hydroxyzine promethazine
antianginals:	amyl nitrite nitroglycerin nitropaste
synthetic analgesics:	butorphanol nalbuphine pentazocine
steroids:	dexamethasone hydrocortisone methylprednisolone
antiarrhythmics:	bretylium edrophonium lidocaine procainamide propranolol verapamil
hormones:	insulin glucagon oxytocin

3

EMERGENCY IV FLUIDS

TABLE 3.1. APPROXIMATE IONIC CONCENTRATIONS

	IONIC CONC	
	Sodium	*Potassium*
5% Dextrose Injection, USP	0	0
10% Dextrose Injection, USP	0	0
0.9% Sodium Chloride Injection, USP	154	0
Sodium Lactate Injection, USP (M/6 Sodium Lactate)	167	0
2.5% Dextrose & 0.45% Sodium Chloride Injection, USP	77	0
5% Dextrose & 0.2% Sodium Chloride Injection, USP	34	0
5% Dextrose & 0.33% Sodium Chloride Injection, USP	56	0
5% Dextrose & 0.45% Sodium Chloride Injection, USP	77	0
5% Dextrose & 0.9% Sodium Chloride Injection, USP	154	0
10% Dextrose & 0.9% Sodium Chloride Injection, USP	154	0
Ringer's Injection, USP	147.5	4
Lactated Ringer's Injection, USP	130	4
5% Dextrose in Ringer's Injection	147.5	4
Lactated Ringer's with 5% Dextrose	130	4

(mEq/l) AND CALORIES PER LITER					
ENTRATIONS (mEq/l)					
Calcium	*Chloride*	*Lactate*	*Calories per liter*	*OSMOLARITY* (m0sm/l)*	*pH Range*
0	0	0	170	252	3.5-6.5
0	0	0	340	505	3.5-6.5
0	154	0	0	308	4.5-7.0
0	0	167	54	334	6.0-7.3
0	77	0	85	280	3.5-6.0
0	34	0	170	321	3.5-6.0
0	56	0	170	365	3.5-6.0
0	77	0	170	406	3.5-6.0
0	154	0	170	560	3.5-6.0
0	154	0	340	813	3.5-6.0
4.5	156	0	0	309	5.0-7.5
3	109	28	9	273	6.0-7.5
4.5	156	0	170	561	3.5-6.5
3	109	28	180	525	4.0-6.5

Normal physiologic isotonicity range is approximately 280-310 mOsm/liter. Adminis-ration of substantially hypotonic solutions may cause hemolysis and administration f substantially hypertonic solutions may cause vein damage.
dapted from Travenol Laboratories, Inc., Deerfield, Illinois)

PLASMA PROTEIN FRACTION (Plasmanate®)

class:	Protein colloid
actions:	Plasma volume expander
indications:	Hypovolemic states (especially burn shock)
contraindications:	None when used in the management of life-threatening situations
precautions:	Hypertension Short shelf life
side effects:	Edema
dosage:	Dosage should be titrated according to patient's hemodynamic response. Follow accepted resuscitation formulas in the management of burn shock.
route:	IV infusion
pediatric dosage:	Same as given above for adult

DEXTRAN

class:	Imitation protein (sugar) colloid
actions:	Plasma volume expander
indications:	Hypovolemic shock
contraindications:	Patients with known hypersensitivity to the drug Patients receiving anticoagulants
precautions:	Severe anaphylactic reactions have been known to occur Monitor for circulatory overload Can impede accurate blood typing as dextran molecule coats the erythrocytes
side effects:	Nausea Vomiting
dosage:	Dosage should be titrated according to patient's hemodynamic response
route:	IV infusion
pediatric dosage:	Same as given above for adult

HETASTARCH (Hespan®)

class:	Artificial colloid
actions:	Plasma volume expander
indications:	Hypovolemic shock
contraindications:	Patients receiving anticoagulants
precautions:	Monitor for circulatory overload Large volumes of hetastarch may alter the coagulation mechanism
side effects:	Nausea Vomiting
dosage:	Dosage should be titrated according to patient's hemodynamic response
route:	IV infusion
pediatric dosage:	No data available pertaining to use in children

LACTATED RINGER'S

class: Isotonic crystalloid

actions: Approximates the electrolyte concentration of the blood

indications: Hypovolemic shock

contraindications: Congestive heart failure
Renal failure

precautions: Monitor for circulatory overload

side effects: Rare

dosage: *Hypovolemic shock* (systolic less than 90 mm/Hg). Infuse 'wide open' until a systolic of 100 mm/Hg is attained.
Once a systolic of 100 mm/Hg has been attained then infusion should be slowed to 100 ml/hour.
Other: As indicated by the patient condition and situation being treated

route: IV infusion

pediatric dosage: Same as adult

5% DEXTROSE IN WATER (D_5W)

class:	Sugar solution
actions:	Glucose nutrient solution
indications:	IV access for emergency drugs For dilution of concentrated drugs for IV infusion
contraindications:	Should not be used as a fluid replacement for hypovolemic states
precautions:	Monitor for circulatory overload Draw tube of blood before administering to diabetics
side effects:	Rare
dosage:	Generally administered to keep open (TKO)
route:	IV infusion
pediatric dosage:	Same as adult

10% DEXTROSE IN WATER ($D_{10}W$)

class:	Hypertonic sugar solution
actions:	Replaces blood glucose
indications:	Hypoglycemia Neonatal resuscitation
contraindications:	Should not be used as fluid replacement for hypovolemic states
precautions:	Monitor for circulatory overload Draw tube of blood before administering $D_{10}W$ to diabetics
side effects:	Rare
dosage:	Dependent upon patient condition and condition being treated
route:	IV infusion
pediatric dosage:	Same as above

0.9% SODIUM CHLORIDE (Normal Saline)

class:	Isotonic electrolyte
actions:	Fluid and sodium replacement
indications:	Heat-related problems (e.g., heat exhaustion, heat stroke) Freshwater drowning Hypovolemia Diabetic ketoacidosis
contraindications:	Congestive heart failure
precautions:	Electrolyte depletion (K^+, Mg^{++}, Ca^{++}, among others) can occur following administration of large amounts of normal saline
side effects:	Thirst
dosage:	Dependent upon patient condition and situation being treated. In freshwater drowning and heat emergencies, the administration is usually rapid.
route:	IV infusion
pediatric dosage:	Dose is dependent on patient size and condition

0.45% SODIUM CHLORIDE
(1/2 Normal Saline)

class:	Hypotonic electrolyte
actions:	Slow rehydration
indications:	Patients with diminished renal and/or cardiovascular function where rapid rehydration is not indicated
contraindications:	Cases where rapid rehydration is indicated
precautions:	Electrolyte depletion can occur following administration of large amounts of 1/2 normal saline
side effects:	Rare
dosage:	Dependent upon patient condition and situation being treated
route:	IV infusion
pediatric dosage:	Dose is based upon patient size and condition

5% DEXTROSE IN 0.9% SODIUM CHLORIDE (D_5NS)

class:	Hypertonic sugar and electrolyte solution
actions:	Provides electrolyte and sugar replacement
indications:	Heat-related disorders Freshwater drowning Hypovolemia Peritonitis
contraindications:	Should not be administered to patients with impaired renal and/or cardiovascular function
precautions:	Draw tube of blood before administering to diabetics
side effects:	Rare
dosage:	Dependent upon patient condition and situation being treated
route:	IV infusion
pediatric dosage:	Dose is dependent upon patient size and condition

5% DEXTROSE IN 0.45% SODIUM CHLORIDE (D_5½NS)

class:	Slightly hypertonic sugar and electrolyte solution
action:	Provides electrolyte and sugar replacement
indications:	Heat exhaustion Diabetic disorders For use as a "TKO" solution in patients with impaired renal and/or cardiovascular function
contraindications:	Situations where rapid fluid replacement is indicated
precautions:	Draw tube of blood before administering to diabetics
side effects:	Rare
dosage:	Dependent upon patient condition and situation being treated
route:	IV infusion
pediatric dosage:	Dose is dependent upon patient size and condition

5% DEXTROSE IN LACTATED RINGER'S (D_5LR)

class:	Hypertonic sugar and electrolyte solution
actions:	Provides electrolyte and sugar replacement
indications:	Hypovolemic shock Hemorrhagic shock Certain cases of acidosis
contraindications:	Should not be administered to patients with decreased renal and/or cardiovascular function
precautions:	Monitor for signs of circulatory overload Draw tube of blood before administering to diabetics
side effects:	Rare
dosage:	Dependent upon patient condition and situation being treated
route:	IV infusion
pediatric dosage:	Dose is dependent upon patient size and condition

4

PEDIATRIC EMERGENCY DRUGS

SPECIAL CONSIDERATIONS: PEDIATRICS

The administration of life-saving medications to children presents several problems to emergency personnel. First, it is essential to accurately estimate the child's weight in kilograms. The majority of the pediatric drug dosages are calculated based upon the child's weight. Overestimation of body weight can lead to overdosage of the drug. Underestimation can cause less than therapeutic levels of the drug within the blood. Second, the drug dosages are often so small that dilution of the drug is often required. Finally, the physical size of the child sometimes makes administration difficult.

The pediatric drug dosages for the most commonly prescribed emergency drugs have been presented in Chapter 1, Quick Drug Reference. The drugs in this section have been broken down and the dosage listed by specific patient weights. This will facilitate easy and rapid reference when confronted by a pediatric patient requiring pharmacological intervention.

how to use this section

1. *Estimate the patient's weight* (often a fairly reliable weight can be obtained from the parents—or refer to page 97).
2. *Convert the patient's weight to kilograms using the Conversion Table* on pages 98 to 99.
3. Consult the Drug Dosage chart beginning on page 100 and *select the column which is closest to the patient's actual weight*. The drug dosages for that weight are provided.

AVERAGE WEIGHT/AGE FOR PEDIATRIC PATIENTS

age	*weight(lb)*	*weight(kg)*
Birth	7	3.5
3 mo	10	5
6 mo	15	7
9 mo	18	8
1 yr	22	10
2 yr	26	12
3 yr	33	15
4 yr	37	17
5 yr	40	18
6 yr	44	20
7 yr	50	23
8 yr	56	25
9 yr	60	28
10 yr	70	33
11 yr	75	35
12 yr	85	40
13 yr	98	44

(*From* Walraven G: Manual of Advanced Prehospital Care. Robert J. Brady Co., Bowie, Maryland, 1978)

CONVERSION TABLE

lbs →	kgs
2.2	1
4.4	2
6.6	3
8.8	4
11	5
13.2	6
15.4	7
17.6	8
19.8	9
22	10
24.2	11
26.4	12
28.6	13
30.8	14
33	15
35.2	16
37.4	17
39.6	18
41.8	19
44	20
46.2	21

lbs →	kgs
48.4	22
50.6	23
52.8	24
55	25
57.2	26
59.4	27
61.6	28
63.8	29
66	30
68.2	31
70.4	32
72.6	33
74.8	34
77	35
79.2	36
81.4	37
83.6	38
85.8	39
88	40
90.2	41
92.4	42

lbs →	*kgs*
94.6	43
96.8	44
99	45
101.2	46
103.4	47
105.6	48
107.8	49
110	50
112.2	51
114.4	52
116.6	53
118.8	54
121	55
123.2	56
125.4	57
127.6	58
129.8	59
132	60
134.2	61
136.4	62
138.6	63
140.8	64
142	65
144.2	66

lbs →	*kgs*
146.4	67
148.6	68
150.8	69
154	70
156.2	71
158.4	72
160.6	73
162.8	74
165	75
167.2	76
169.4	77
171.6	78
173.8	79
176	80
178.2	81
180.4	82
182.6	83
184.8	84
187	85
189.2	86
191.4	87
193.6	88
195.8	89
198	90

DRUG DOSAGE CHART

body weight (kg)

	1	*2*	*3*	*4*	*5*
Atropine Sulfate	0.02 mg	0.04 mg	0.06 mg	0.08 mg	0.10 mg
Benadryl®	1 mg	2 mg	3 mg	4 mg	5 mg
Calcium Chloride	20 mg	40 mg	60 mg	80 mg	100 mg
Decadron®	0.3 mg	0.6 mg	0.9 mg	1.2 mg	1.5 mg
Dextrose 50%	0.5 gm	1.0 gm	1.5 gm	2.0 gm	2.5 gm
Dopamine®	5 μg/min	10 μg/min	15 μg/min	20 μg/min	25 μg/min
Epinephrine 1:10,000	0.01 mg	0.02 mg	0.03 mg	0.04 mg	0.05 mg
Hyperstat®	5 mg	10 mg	15 mg	20 mg	25 mg

1 to 5 kilograms

body weight (kg)

	1	2	3	4	5
Inderal®	0.01 mg	0.02 mg	0.03 mg	0.04 mg	0.05 mg
Isuprel®	0.1 μg/min	0.2 μg/min	0.3 μg/min	0.4 μg/min	0.5 μg/min
Lasix®	1 mg	2 mg	3 mg	4 mg	5 mg
Lidocaine Bolus	1 mg	2 mg	3 mg	4 mg	5 mg
Lidocaine Infusion	30 μg/min	60 μg/min	90 μg/min	120 μg/min	150 μg/min
Narcan®	0.01 mg	0.02 mg	0.03 mg	0.04 mg	0.05 mg
Phenergan®	0.5 mg	1.0 mg	1.5 mg	2.0 mg	2.5 mg
Sodium Bicarbonate	1 mEq	2 mEq	3 mEq	4 mEq	5 mEq
Verapamil	0.1 mg	0.2 mg	0.3 mg	0.4 mg	0.5 mg

	body weight (kg)				
	6	**7**	**8**	**9**	**10**
Atropine Sulfate	0.12 mg	0.14 mg	0.16 mg	0.18 mg	0.20 mg
Benadryl®	6 mg	7 mg	8 mg	9 mg	10 mg
Calcium Chloride	120 mg	140 mg	160 mg	180 mg	200 mg
Decadron®	1.8 mg	2.1 mg	2.4 mg	2.7 mg	3.0 mg
Dextrose 50%	3.0 gm	3.5 gm	4.0 gm	4.5 gm	5.0 gm
Dopamine®	30 μg/min	35 μg/min	40 μg/min	45 μg/min	50 μg/min
Epinephrine 1:10,000	0.06 mg	0.07 mg	0.08 mg	0.09 mg	0.1 mg
Hyperstat®	30 mg	35 mg	40 mg	45 mg	50 mg

Drug Dosage Chart (continued)

6 to 10 kilograms

	body weight (kg)				
	6	**7**	**8**	**9**	**10**
Inderal®	0.06 mg	0.07 mg	0.08 mg	0.09 mg	0.1 mg
Isuprel®	0.6 μg/min	0.7 μg/min	0.8 μg/min	0.9 μg/min	1 μg/min
Lasix®	6 mg	7 mg	8 mg	9 mg	10 mg
Lidocaine Bolus	6 mg	7 mg	8 mg	9 mg	10 mg
Lidocaine Infusion	180 μg/min	210 μg/min	240 μg/min	270 μg/min	300 μg/min
Narcan®	0.06 mg	0.07 mg	0.08 mg	0.09 mg	0.10 mg
Phenergan®	3 mg	3.5 mg	4 mg	4.5 mg	5 mg
Sodium Bicarbonate	6 mEq	7 mEq	8 mEq	9 mEq	10 mEq
Verapamil®	0.6 mg	0.7 mg	0.8 mg	0.9 mg	1.0 mg

11 to 15 kilograms

	body weight (kg)				
	11	**12**	**13**	**14**	**15**
Atropine Sulfate	0.22 mg	0.24 mg	0.26 mg	0.28 mg	0.3 mg
Benadryl®	11 mg	12 mg	13 mg	14 mg	15 mg
Calcium Chloride	220 mg	240 mg	260 mg	280 mg	300 mg
Decadron®	3.3 mg	3.7 mg	4.0 mg	4.3 mg	4.6 mg
Dextrose 50%	5.5 gm	6.0 gm	6.5 gm	7.0 gm	7.5 gm
Dopamine®	55 μg/min	60 μg/min	65 μg/min	70 μg/min	75 μg/min
Epinephrine 1:10,000	0.11 mg	0.12 mg	0.13 mg	0.14 mg	0.15 mg
Hyperstat®	55 mg	60 mg	65 mg	70 mg	75 mg

	body weight (kg)				
	11	**12**	**13**	**14**	**15**
Inderal®	0.11 mg	0.12 mg	0.13 mg	0.14 mg	0.15 mg
Isuprel®	1.1 μg/min	1.2 μg/min	1.3 μg/min	1.4 μg/min	1.5 μg/min
Lasix®	11 mg	12 mg	13 mg	14 mg	15 mg
Lidocaine Bolus	11 mg	12 mg	13 mg	14 mg	15 mg
Lidocaine Infusion	330 μg/min	360 μg/min	390 μg/min	420 μg/min	450 μg/min
Narcan®	0.11 mg	0.12 mg	0.13 mg	0.14 mg	0.15 mg
Phenergan®	5.5 mg	6.0 mg	6.5 mg	7.0 mg	7.5 mg
Sodium Bicarbonate	11 mEq	12 mEq	13 mEq	14 mEq	15 mEq
Verapamil®	1.1 mg	1.2 mg	1.3 mg	1.4 mg	1.5 mg

	body weight (kg)				
	16	**17**	**18**	**19**	**20**
Atropine Sulfate	0.32 mg	0.34 mg	0.36 mg	0.38 mg	0.4 mg
Benadryl®	16 mg	17 mg	18 mg	19 mg	20 mg
Calcium Chloride	320 mg	340 mg	360 mg	380 mg	400 mg
Decadron®	4.9 mg	5.0 mg	5.0 mg	5.0 mg	5.0 mg
Dextrose 50%	8.0 gm	8.5 gm	9.0 gm	9.5 gm	10 gm
Dopamine®	80 μg/min	85 μg/min	90 μg/min	95 μg/min	100 μg/min
Epinephrine 1:10,000	0.16 mg	0.17 mg	0.18 mg	0.19 mg	0.2 mg
Hyperstat®	80 mg	85 mg	90 mg	95 mg	100 mg

16 to 20 kilograms

	body weight (kg)				
	16	**17**	**18**	**19**	**20**
Inderal®	0.16 mg	0.17 mg	0.18 mg	0.19 mg	0.20 mg
Isuprel®	1.6 μg/min	1.7 μg/min	1.8 μg/min	1.9 μg/min	2.0 μg/min
Lasix®	16 mg	17 mg	18 mg	19 mg	20 mg
Lidocaine Bolus	16 mg	17 mg	18 mg	19 mg	20 mg
Lidocaine Infusion	0.48 mg/min	0.51 mg/min	0.54 mg/min	0.57 mg/min	0.6 mg/min
Narcan®	0.16 mg	0.17 mg	0.18 mg	0.19 mg	0.2 mg
Phenergan®	8.0 mg	8.5 mg	9.0 mg	9.5 mg	10 mg
Sodium Bicarbonate	16 mEq	17 mEq	18 mEq	19 mEq	20 mEq
Verapamil®	1.6 mg	1.7 mg	1.8 mg	1.9 mg	2. mg

Drug Dosage Chart (continued)

	body weight (kg)				
	21	**22**	**23**	**24**	**25**
Atropine Sulfate	0.42 mg	0.44 mg	0.46 mg	0.48 mg	0.5 mg
Benadryl®	21 mg	22 mg	23 mg	24 mg	25 mg
Calcium Chloride	420 mg	440 mg	460 mg	480 mg	500 mg
Decadron®	5 mg	5 mg	5 mg	5 mg	5 mg
Dextrose 50%	10.5 gm	11.0 gm	11.5 gm	12.0 gm	12.5 gm
Dopamine®	105 μg/min	110 μg/min	115 μg/min	120 μg/min	125 μg/min
Epinephrine 1:10,000	0.21 mg	0.22 mg	0.23 mg	0.24 mg	0.25 mg
Hyperstat®	105 mg	110 mg	115 mg	120 mg	125 mg

	body weight (kg)				
	21	**22**	**23**	**24**	**25**
Inderal®	0.21 mg	0.22 mg	0.23 mg	0.24 mg	0.25 mg
Isuprel®	2.1 μg/min	2.2 μg/min	2.3 μg/min	2.4 μg/min	2.5 μg/min
Lasix®	21 mg	22 mg	23 mg	24 mg	25 mg
Lidocaine Bolus	21 mg	22 mg	23 mg	24 mg	25 mg
Lidocaine Infusion	0.63 mg/min	0.66 mg/min	0.69 mg/min	0.72 mg/min	0.75 mg/min
Narcan®	0.21 mg	0.22 mg	0.23 mg	0.24 mg	0.25 mg
Phenergan®	10.5 mg	11.0 mg	11.5 mg	12.0 mg	12.5 mg
Sodium Bicarbonate	21 mEq	22 mEq	23 mEq	24 mEq	25 mEq
Verapamil®	2.1 mg	2.2 mg	2.3 mg	2.4 mg	2.5 mg

	body weight (kg)				
	26	**27**	**28**	**29**	**30**
Atropine Sulfate	0.5 mg	0.5 mg	0.5 mg	0.5 mg	0.5 mg
Benadryl®	26 mg	27 mg	28 mg	29 mg	30 mg
Calcium Chloride	500 mg	500 mg	500 mg	500 mg	500 mg
Decadron®	5 mg	5 mg	5 mg	5 mg	5 mg
Dextrose 50%	13.0 gm	13.5 gm	14.0 gm	14.5 gm	15.0 gm
Dopamine®	130 μg/min	135 μg/min	140 μg/min	145 μg/min	150 μg/min
Epinephrine 1:10,000	0.26 mg	0.27 mg	0.28 mg	0.29 mg	0.30 mg
Hyperstat®	130 mg	135 mg	140 mg	145 mg	150 mg

	body weight (kg)				
	26	**27**	**28**	**29**	**30**
Inderal®	0.26 mg	0.27 mg	0.28 mg	0.29 mg	0.30 mg
Isuprel®	2.6 μg/min	2.7 μg/min	2.8 μg/min	2.9 μg/min	3.0 μg/min
Lasix®	26 mg	27 mg	28 mg	29 mg	30 mg
Lidocaine Bolus	26 mg	27 mg	28 mg	29 mg	30 mg
Lidocaine Infusion	0.78 mg/min	0.81 mg/min	0.84 mg/min	0.87 mg/min	0.9 mg/min
Narcan®	0.26 mg	0.27 mg	0.28 mg	0.29 mg	0.30 mg
Phenergan®	13.0 mg	13.5 mg	14.0 mg	14.5 mg	15.0 mg
Sodium Bicarbonate	26 mEq	27 mEq	28 mEq	29 mEq	30 mEq
Verapamil®	2.6 mg	2.7 mg	2.8 mg	2.9 mg	3.0 mg

body weight (kg)

	31	***32***	***33***	***34***	***35***
Atropine Sulfate	5.0 mg	5.0 mg	5.0 mg	5.0 mg	5.0 mg
Benadryl®	31 mg	32 mg	33 mg	34 mg	35 mg
Calcium Chloride	500 mg	500 mg	500 mg	500 mg	500 mg
Decadron®	5 mg	5 mg	5 mg	5 mg	5 mg
Dextrose 50%	15.5 gm	16.0 gm	16.5 gm	17.0 gm	17.5 gm
Dopamine®	155 μg/min	160 μg/min	165 μg/min	170 μg/min	175 μg/min
Epinephrine 1:10,000	0.31 mg	0.32 mg	0.33 mg	0.34 mg	0.35 mg
Hyperstat®	155 mg	160 mg	165 mg	170 mg	175 mg

	body weight (kg)				
	31	**32**	**33**	**34**	**35**
Inderal®	0.31 mg	0.32 mg	0.33 mg	0.34 mg	0.35 mg
Isuprel®	3.1 μg/min	3.2 μg/min	3.3 μg/min	3.4 μg/min	3.5 μg/min
Lasix®	31 mg	32 mg	33 mg	34 mg	35 mg
Lidocaine Bolus	31 mg	32 mg	33 mg	34 mg	35 mg
Lidocaine Infusion	0.93 mg/min	0.96 mg/min	0.99 mg/min	1.02 mg/min	1.05 mg/min
Narcan®	0.31 mg	0.32 mg	0.33 mg	0.34 mg	0.35 mg
Phenergan®	15.5 mg	16.0 mg	16.5 mg	17.0 mg	17.5 mg
Sodium Bicarbonate	31 mEq	32 mEq	33 mEq	34 mEq	35 mEq
Verapamil®	3.0 mg	3.0 mg	3.0 mg	3.0 mg	3.0 mg

	body weight (kg)				
	36	**37**	**38**	**39**	**40**
Atropine Sulfate	0.5 mg	0.5 mg	0.5 mg	0.5 mg	0.5 mg
Benadryl®	36 mg	37 mg	38 mg	39 mg	40 mg
Calcium Chloride	500 mg	500 mg	500 mg	500 mg	500 mg
Decadron®	5 mg	5 mg	5 mg	5 mg	5 mg
Dextrose 50%	18.0 gm	18.5 gm	19.0 gm	19.5 gm	20.0 gm
Dopamine®	180 μg/min	185 μg/min	190 μg/min	195 μg/min	200 μg/min
Epinephrine 1:10,000	0.36 mg	0.37 mg	0.38 mg	0.39 mg	0.40 mg
Hyperstat®	180 mg	185 mg	190 mg	195 mg	200 mg

	body weight (kg)				
	36	**37**	**38**	**39**	**40**
Inderal®	0.36 mg	0.37 mg	0.38 mg	0.39 mg	0.4 mg
Isuprel®	3.6 μg/min	3.7 μg/min	3.8 μg/min	3.9 μg/min	4.0 μg/min
Lasix®	36 mg	37 mg	38 mg	39 mg	40 mg
Lidocaine Bolus	36 mg	37 mg	38 mg	39 mg	40 mg
Lidocaine Infusion	1.1 mg/min	1.1 mg/min	1.1 mg/min	1.2 mg/min	1.2 mg/min
Narcan®	0.36 mg	0.37 mg	0.38 mg	0.39 mg	0.4 mg
Phenergan®	18 mg	18.5 mg	19 mg	19.5 mg	20 mg
Sodium Bicarbonate	36 mEq	37 mEq	38 mEq	39 mEq	40 mEq
Verapamil®	3 mg	3 mg	3 mg	3 mg	3 mg

5

HOME MEDICATION REFERENCE GUIDE

HOME MEDICATION CLASSES

class	*actions*
Analgesics	Raises pain threshold Alleviates anxiety and fear Alters physiological response to pain
Anorexiants	Controls appetite
Antacids	Reduce stomach and duodenal activity Raises stomach pH
Antianginals	Dilates peripheral and coronary arterioles
Antiarrhythmics	Suppresses ectopic activity Controls rhythm of heart
Antiarthritics	Controls joint inflammation and pain associated with arthritis
Antibiotics	Combats microorganisms
Anticoagulants	Prolongs blood clotting time
Anticholinergics	Blocks actions of acetylcholine thus potentiating sympathetic nervous system
Anticonvulsants	Suppresses seizure activity in the brain Suppresses spread of seizure activity in motor cortex

class	*actions*
Antidepressants	Tricyclic compounds potentiate sympathetic effects by preventing the uptake of norepinephrine in the CNS Monoamine oxidase (MAO) inhibitors prevent impulse transmission at the neurons and inhibit catecholamine breakdown
Antidiarrheal	Reduces bowel motility
Antiemetic	Relieves or prevents nausea and/or vomiting Stimulates H_2 histamine receptors
Antihistamines	Blocks release of histamine
Antihypertensives	Lowers blood pressure by sympathetic blockade Causes peripheral vasodilation
Antipsychotics	Phenothiazines are thought to block dopamine receptors in the brain associated with mood and behavior
Antispasmodics	Relieves pain Blocks acetylcholine in parts of the parasympathetic nervous system
Antituberculosis	Deactivates the tubercle bacillus
Bronchodilators	Relaxes smooth muscle of bronchioles
Cardiac Glycosides	Increases cardiac output Slows SA and AV conduction

class	*actions*
	Positive inotrope Controls certain rhythm disorders
Diuretics	Stimulates release of water and sodium chloride from kidneys Inhibits reabsorpiton of sodium in nephron
Hypnotics and Sedatives	Induces sleep Depresses CNS
Hypoglycemics	Provides insulin to promote uptake of glucose by the cells
Laxatives and Stool Softeners	Stimulates peristalsis Alters fecal consistency
Steroids	Controls inflammatory response
Sulfamides	Antibiotics for UTI (urinary tract infections)
Tranquilizers	Induces calmness without depression of level of consciousness Depresses CNS

COMMON HOME MEDICATIONS

The following section contains a listing of over 1,100 of the most commonly prescribed medications. Generic names are listed in BOLD TYPE. If additional information is required concerning a drug, the *Physician's Desk Reference* or similar source should be consulted.

drug	*usage*
A.P.C. WITH CODEINE	Narcotic Analgesic/Cough Suppressant
A.S.A. and Codeine	Aspirin/Narcotic
A.S.A.	Aspirin
A.S.A. Enseals	Aspirin
A-M-T	Aluminum/ Magnesium Antacid
A-Poxide	Tranquilizer
A'Cenol	Acetaminophen Analgesic
Accurbron	Xanthine Bronchodilator
Aceta	Acetaminophen Analgesic
Aceta with Codeine	Acetaminophen/ Narcotic Analgesic

drug	*usage*
ACETAMINOPHEN	Analgesic
ACETAZOLAMIDE	Mild Diuretic (Carbonic Anhydrase Inhibitor)
Achromycin	Antibiotic
Actamin	Acetaminophen Analgesic
Actamine Tablets	Antihistamine/ Decongestant
Actifed Tablets	Antihistamine/ Decongestant
Actifed-C Expectorant	Decongestant/ Narcotic
Actrapid	Insulin
Adapin	Antidepressant (Tricyclic)
Adipex	Nonamphetamine Appetite Suppressant
Adphen	Nonamphetamine Appetite Suppressant
Aerolate	Xanthine Bronchodilator
Afko-Lube Lax	Laxative
Afrin	Nasal Decongestant

drug	*usage*
Afrinol Repetabs	Bronchodilator/ Decongestant
AK-ZOL	Mild Diuretic (Carbonic Anhydrase Inhibitor)
Aldactazide	Diuretic
Aldactone	Diuretic
Aldomet	Antihypertensive
Aldoril	Antihypertensive
Alermine	Antihistamine
Algenic Alka	Aluminum/ Magnesium Antacid
Algimate	Aluminum/ Magnesium Antacid
Algitab	Aluminum/ Magnesium Antacid
Alka-Med	Aluminum/ Magnesium Antacid
Alka-Seltzer	Effervescent Antacid
Alka-2	Calcium Antacid
Alkets Calcium	Calcium Antacid

drug	*usage*
ALLOPURINOL	Anti-Gout
Almacone	Aluminum/ Magnesium/ Simethicone Antacid
ALPRAZOLAM	Tranquilizer
AlternaGel	Aluminum Antacid
Alu-Cap	Aluminum Antacid
Alu-Tab	Aluminum Antacid
Aludrox	Aluminum/ Magnesium Antacid
Alumid	Aluminum/ Magnesium Antacid
Alumid Plus	Aluminum/ Magnesium/ Simethicone Antacid
Aluminum Hydroxide Gel	Aluminum Antacid
Alupent	Bronchodilator
Alurex	Aluminum/ Magnesium Antacid
Aluscop	Aluminum/ Magnesium Antacid

drug	***usage***
Alusil	Aluminum/ Magnesium Antacid
Ambenyl Expectorant	Cough Suppressant/ Expectorant
Amcill	Penicillin Type Antibiotic
Amen	Female Hormone
Ameri-EZP	Urinary Anti-infective
Amitone	Calcium Antacid
Amitril	Antidepressant (Tricyclic)
AMITRIPTYLINE	Antidepressant (Tricyclic)
AMOBARBITOL	Hypnotic/Sedative/ Anticonvulsant
AMOXAPINE	Antidepressant (Tricyclic)
AMOXICILLIN	Penicillin Type Antibiotic
Amoxil	Penicillin Type Antibiotic
Amphenol	Acetaminophen Analgesic
Amphojel	Aluminum Antacid

drug	*usage*
AMPICILLIN	Penicillin Type Antibiotic
Ampico	Penicillin Type Antibiotic
Anaprox	Nonsteroid Anti-inflammatory
Android	Male Hormone
Ang-O-Span	Antianginal
Anorex	Nonamphetamine Appetite Suppressant
Antalgesic	Aspirin
Antar	Aluminum/ Magnesium/ Simethicine Antacid
Antipress	Antidepressant (Tricyclic)
Antivert	Antiemetic/ Antivertigo
Anuphen	Acetaminophen Analgesic
APAP	Acetaminophen Analgesic
Apresazide	Antihypertensive
Apresoline	Antihypertensive

drug	***usage***
Aptrol	Nonamphetamine Appetite Suppressant
Aquaphyllin	Xanthine Bronchodilator
Aquatensen	Diuretic
Artane	Anticholinergic
Ascriptin	Aspirin
Asendin	Antidepressant (Tricyclic)
Asmalix	Xanthine Bronchodilator
Asperbuf	Aspirin
Atarax	Antihistamine/ Antinausea/ Antianxiety
ATENOLOL	Beta Blocker
Athrombin-K	Anticoagulant
Ativan	Tranquilizer
Atromid-S	Antihyperlipidemic (reduces blood lipids)
Aventyl	Antidepressant (Tricyclic)
AZATADINE MALEATE	Antihistamine
Azene	Tranquilizer

drug	usage
Azo Gantrisin	Urinary Antibiotic
Azo-Standard	Urinary Analgesic
Azo-Sulfisoxazole	Urinary Antibiotic
Azo-Sulfizin	Urinary Antibiotic
Azo-100	Urinary Analgesic
Azodine	Urinary Analgesic
Azolid	Anti-inflammatory
Azulfidine	Sulfonamide
Bacarate	Nonamphetamine Appetite Suppressant
Bactrim	Urinary Antibiotic
Bamate	Tranquilizer
Barbipil	Hypnotic/Sedative/ Anticonvulsant
Barbita	Hypnotic/Sedative/ Anticonvulsant
Basaljel	Aluminum Antacid
Bactocill	Antibiotic
Bayapap with Codeine	Acetaminophen/ Narcotic Analgesic
BECLOMETHASONE	Steroid
Beclovent	Steroid
Beepen-VK	Antibiotic (Penicillin)

drug	*usage*
Bell/ans	Sodium Bicarbonate Antacid
Benachlor	Antihistamine
Benadryl	Antihistamine
Bendectin	Antiemetic
Bendopa	Anti-Parkinsonian
Bendylate	Antihistamine
Bentomine	Gastrointestinal Anticholinergic Agent
Bentyl	Gastrointestinal Anticholinergic Agent
Bentyl w/ Phenobarbitol	Gastrointestinal Anticholinergic Agent
BENZPHETAMINE HCl	Amphetamine
BENZTROPINE MESYLATE	Anticholinergic
Bisodol	Aluminum/ Calcium Antacid
Bisodol Powder	Effervescent Antacid
Blocadren Tablets	Beta Blocker
Bonine	Antiemetic/ Antivertigo

drug	*usage*
Bontril PDM	Nonamphetamine Appetite Suppressant
Brethine	Bronchodilator
Brevicon	Contraceptive
Bricanyl	Bronchodilator
Bristacycline	Antibiotic
Bristamycin	Antibiotic
Bromamine	Antihistamine
Bromatane	Antihistamine
Bromo Seltzer	Effervescent Analgesic
Bromophen	Antihistamine/ Decongestant
Bromphen	Antihistamine
BROMPHENIRAMINE MALEATE	Antihistamine
Bronkodyl	Xanthine Bronchodilator
Bu-Lax Plus	Laxative
Buffaprin	Aspirin
BUTABARBITAL	Hypnotic/Sedative/ Anticonvulsant
Butal	Hypnotic/Sedative/ Anticonvulsant

drug	*usage*
Butalan	Hypnotic/Sedative/ Anticonvulsant
Butatran	Hypnotic/Sedative/ Anticonvulsant
Butazem	Hypnotic/Sedative/ Anticonvulsant
Butazolidin	Anti-inflammatory
Buticaps	Hypnotic/Sedative/ Anticonvulsant
Butisol Sodium	Hypnotic/Sedative/ Anticonvulsant
Calan	Calcium-ion Antagonist (Antianginal)
Calcilac	Calcium Antacid
Calcium Carbonate	Calcium Antacid
Calglycine	Calcium Antacid
Cam-Ap-Es	Antihypertensive
Camalox	Aluminum/ Calcium/ Magnesium Antacid
Capital with Codeine	Acetaminophen/ Narcotic Analgesic
Capoten	Antihypertensive
CAPTOPRIL	Antihypertensive

drug	***usage***
Carafate	Anti-Ulcer
Carbrital	Hypnotic/Sedative
CARISOPRODOL	Skeletal Muscle Relaxant
Catapres	Antihypertensive
Ceclor	Antibiotic
CEFACLOR	Antibiotic
Cenafed	Bronchodilator/ Decongestant
Centet-250	Antibiotic
Centrax	Tranquilizer
CEPHALEXIN	Antibiotic
CEPHRADINE	Antibiotic
Cerespan	Vasodilator
Chlo-Amine	Antihistamine
Chlor-Mal	Antihistamine
Chlor-Niramine	Antihistamine
CHLORAL HYDRATE	Sedative/Hypnotic
Chloramate Unicelles	Antihistamine
Chloramead	Phenothiazine Tranquilizer
Chlordiazachel	Tranquilizer
CHLORDIAZEPOXIDE	Tranquilizer

drug	*usage*
Chlorofon-F	Skeletal Muscle Relaxant
Chlorophen	Antihistamine
CHLOROTHIAZIDE	Diuretic
CHLORPHENESIN CARBAMATE	Skeletal Muscle Relaxant
CHLORPHENIRAMINE MALEATE	Antihistamine
CHLORPROMAZINE	Phenothiazine Tranquilizer
CHLORPROPAMIDE	Antidiabetic
Chlorspan	Antihistamine
Chlortab	Antihistamine
CHLORTHALIDONE	Diuretic
Chlorzide	Diuretic
Chlorzone Forte	Skeletal Muscle Relaxant
Choledyl	Xanthine Bronchodilator
Choloxin	Antihyperlipidemic (Reduces blood lipids)
Chooz	Calcium Antacid
Cibalith	Antipsychotic

drug	*usage*
CIMETIDINE	Anti-Ulcer (H2 Antagonist)
Cin-Quin	Antiarrhythmic
Ciramine	Antihistamine
Citrocarbonate	Effervescent Antacid
Cleocin	Antibiotic
CLINDAMYCIN	Antibiotic
Clinoril	Nonsteroid Anti-inflammatory
CLOFIBRATE	Antihyperlipidemic (Reduces blood lipids)
CLONIDINE	Antihypertensive
CLORAZEPATE	Tranquilizer
Clorazine	Phenothiazine Tranquilizer
Co-Gel	Aluminum/ Calcium/ Magnesium Antacid
Coastaldyne	Acetaminophen/ Narcotic Analgesic
Cocillin-V-K	Antibiotic (Penicillin)
Codap	Acetaminophen/ Narcotic Analgesic

drug	*usage*
CODEINE	Narcotic
Cogentin	Anticholinergic
Cohidrate	Sedative/Hypnotic
Colonaid	Antidiarrheal
Combid	Gastrointestinal Anticholinergic Agent
Combipres	Antihypertensive
Comfolax-plus	Laxative
Compazine	Phenothiazine Anti-Emetic/ Antipsychotic
CONJUGATED ESTROGENS	Female Hormone
Constiban	Laxative
Coprobate	Tranquilizer
Corgard	Beta Blocker
Cortan	Steroid
Coumadin	Anticoagulant
Creamalin	Aluminum/ Magnesium Antacid
Crystodigin	Cardiac Glycoside (Digitalis)
Curretab	Female Hormone
CYCLANDELATE	Vasodilator

drug	*usage*
Cycline-250	Antibiotic
CYCLOBENZAPRINE	Skeletal Muscle Relaxant
Cyclopar 500	Antibiotic
Cyclospasmol	Vasodilator
Cydel	Vasodilator
Cylert	Psychotherapeutic
Cyprodine	Phenothiazine-type Antihistamine
CYPROHEPTADINE HCl	Phenothiazine-type Antihistamine
Cyvaso	Vasodilator
D-Feda	Bronchodilator/ Decongestant
D-S-S plus	Laxative
Dalmane	Sedative/Sleeping Agent
Dapa	Acetaminophen Analgesic
Darvocet-N	Acetaminophen Analgesic
Darvon	Synthetic Narcotic
Darvon Compound	Synthetic Narcotic Analgesic
Datril	Acetaminophen Analgesic

drug	*usage*
De-Tone	Cardiac Glycoside (Digitalis)
Decadron	Steroid
Declomycin	Antibiotic
Decohist	Decongestant/ Antihistamine
Delapav	Vasodilator
Delaxin	Skeletal Muscle Relaxant
Delcid	Aluminum/ Magnesium Antacid
Delcophen	Nonamphetamine Appetite Suppressant
Delta-E	Antibiotic
Deltamycin	Antibiotic
Deltapen-VK	Antibiotic (Penicillin)
Deltasone	Steroid
Demazin	Decongestant/ Antihistamine
DEMECLOCYCLINE	Antibiotic
Demerol	Narcotic
Demulen	Contraceptive
Depakene	Anticonvulsant

drug	*usage*
Depletite	Nonamphetamine Appetite Suppressant
DES	Female Hormone (Estrogen)
DESIPRAMINE	Antidepressant (Tricyclic)
DEXAMETHASONE	Steroid
Dexampex	Amphetamine
DEXCHLORPHENIRAMINE	Antihistamine
Dexedrine	Amphetamine
Dexone	Steroid
DEXTROAMPHETAMINE	Amphetamine
DEXTROTHYROXINE	Antihyperlipidemic (Reduces blood lipids)
Dezone	Steroid
DI-AP-TROL	Nonamphetamine Appetite Suppressant
Di-Azo	Urinary Analgesic
Di-Spaz	Gastrointestinal Anticholinergic Agent
Diabinese	Antidiabetic
Diaction	Antidiarrheal

drug	*usage*
Diahist	Antihistamine
Dialume	Aluminum Antacid
Diamox	Mild Diuretic (Carbonic Anhydrase Inhibitor)
Diaqua	Diuretic
DIAZEPAM	Tranquilizer
Dibent	Gastrointestinal Anticholinergic Agent
Dibent-PB	Gastrointestinal Anticholinergic Agent
Dicarbosil	Calcium Antacid
DICLOXACILLIN	Antibiotic
DICYLOMINE HCl	Gastrointestinal Anticholinergic Agent
Didrez	Amphetamine
Dietaps	Nonamphetamine Appetite Suppressant
DIETHYLPROPION HCl	Nonamphetamine Appetite Suppressant
DIETHYLSTILBESTROL	Female Hormone (Estrogen)

drug	*usage*
DiGel	Aluminum/ Magnesium/ Simethicone Antacid
DIGITOXIN	Cardiac Glycoside (Digitalis)
DIGOXIN	Cardiac Glycoside (Digitalis)
Dilantin	Anticonvulsant
Dilart	Vasodilator
Dilomine	Gastrointestinal Anticholinergic Agent
Dimetane	Antihistamine
Dimetapp Extentabs	Antihistamine/ Decongestant
Diothron	Laxative
Dipav	Vasodilator
Diphen	Antihistamine
Diphenadril	Antihistamine
DIPHENHYDRAMINE HCl	Antihistamine
Diphenylan	Anticonvulsant
DIPYRIDAMOLE	Antianginal
Disanthrol	Laxative
Disophrol Chronotabs	Antihistamine

drug	*usage*
Disophrol Tablets	Antihistamine/ Decongestant
Ditan	Anticonvulsant
Diu-Scrip	Diuretic
Diupres	Antihypertensive
Diuril	Diuretic
Dizmiss	Antiemetic/ Antivertigo
Dolanex	Acetaminophen Analgesic
Dolene	Synthetic Narcotic
Dolene Compound	Synthetic Narcotic Analgesic
Dopar	Anti-Parkinsonian
Doriden	Sedative/Hypnotic
Dormtabs	Sedative/Hypnotic
DOXEPIN HCl	Antidepressant (Tricyclic)
Doxy-C	Antibiotic
Doxychel	Antibiotic
DOXYCYCLINE	Antibiotic
Doxylamine Succinate	Antiemetic
Dralzine	Antihypertensive
Drixoral	Antihistamine/ Decongestant

drug	*usage*
Duration	Nasal Decongestant
Dyazide	Diuretic (Antihypertensive)
Dycill	Antibiotic
Dynapen	Antibiotic
E.E.S.	Antibiotic
E-Mycin	Antibiotic
Ecotrin	Aspirin
El-Da-Mint	Calcium Antacid
Elavil	Antidepressant (Tricyclic)
Eldafed Tablets	Antihistamine/ Decongestant
Eldatapp	Antihistamine/ Decongestant
Elder 65 Compound	Synthetic Narcotic Analgesic
Elixicon	Xanthine Bronchodilator
Elixophyllin	Xanthine Bronchodilator
Empracet with Codeine	Acetaminophen/ Narcotic Analgesic
Empirin	Aspirin
Empirin with Codiene	Aspirin/Narcotic

drug	*usage*
Endep	Antidepressant (Tricyclic)
Enduron	Diuretic
ENO Powder	Effervescent Antacid
Enovid	Contraceptive
Enoxa	Antidiarrheal
Equagesic	Aspirin Analgesic Combination
Equanil	Tranquilizer
Equilet	Calcium Antacid
Eramycin	Antibiotic
ERGOT ALKALOIDS	Antimigraine
Erypar	Antibiotic
Erythrocin	Antibiotic
ERYTHROMYCIN	Antibiotic
Esidrex	Diuretic
Eskalith	Antipsychotic
Estomul-M	Aluminum/ Magnesium Antacid
Estroate	Female Hormone
ETHCHLORVYNOL	Sedative/Hypnotic
Ethril	Antibiotic

drug	*usage*
Eugel	Aluminum/ Calcium/ Magnesium Antacid
Evenol	Tranquilizer
Evestrone	Female Hormone
Ex-Obese	Nonamphetamine Appetite Suppressant
F.M.	Tranquilizer
Fastin	Nonamphetamine Appetite Suppressant
Febrigesic	Acetaminophen Analgesic
Feldene	Non-steroid Anti-inflammatory
FENOPROFEN CALCIUM	Anti-inflammatory
Fenylhist	Antihistamine
Ferndex	Amphetamine
Fernisone	Steroid
Fiorinal	Nonnarcotic analgesic combination
First Sign	Bronchodilator/ Decongestant

drug	*usage*
Flacid	Aluminum/ Magnesium/ Simethicone Antacid
Flagyl	Amoebicide (Trichomonas Infections)
Flexeril	Skeletal Muscle Relaxant
FLUOXYMESTERONE	Male Hormone
FLUPHENAZINE HCl	Phenothiazine Antipsychotic
FLURAZEPAM	Sedative/Sleeping Agent
Forbaxin	Skeletal Muscle Relaxant
Foypromazine	Phenothiazine Tranquilizer
Furadantin	Urinary Antibiotic
Furalan	Urinary Antibiotic
Furan	Urinary Antibiotic
Furatoin	Urinary Antibiotic
FUROSEMIDE	Potent Diuretic
G-1 Tablets	Acetaminophen Analgesic
Gantanol	Urinary Antibiotic

drug	*usage*
Gantrisin	Urinary Antibiotic
Gaviscon	Aluminum/ Magnesium Antacid
Gelusil	Aluminum/ Magnesium/ Simethicone Antacid
Gelusil-M	Aluminum/ Magnesium/ Simethicone Antacid
Glycogel	Aluminum/ Calcium/ Magnesium Antacid
GUANETHIDINE	Antihypertensive
Gustalac	Calcium Antacid
Hal-Chlor	Antihistamine
HALAZEPAM	Tranquilizer
Haldol	Antipsychotic
HALOPERIDOL	Antipsychotic
Halotestin	Male Hormone
Henotal	Hypnotic/Sedative/ Anticonvulsant
Hexadrol	Steroid

drug	***usage***
HHR Tablets	Antihypertensive
Hipprurate	Urinary Antibiotic
Histarall	Antihistamine/ Decongestant
Histaspan	Antihistamine
Histatapp	Antihistamine/ Decongestant
Histex	Antihistamine
Histrey	Antihistamine
HRH Tablets	Antihypertensive
HYDRALAZINE HCl	Antihypertensive
Hydro-Schlor	Diuretic
Hydro-Z	Diuretic
HYDROCHLOROTHIAZIDE	Diuretic
HydroDIURIL	Diuretic
Hydromal	Diuretic
Hydropres	Antihypertensive
HYDROXYZINE HCl	Antihistamine/ Antinausea/ Antianxiety
Hygroton	Diuretic
Hyperetic	Diuretic
Hyserp	Antihypertensive

drug	*usage*
I-PAC	Nonnarcotic analgesic combination
IBUPROFEN	Nonsteroid Anti-inflammatory
Idenal	Nonnarcotic analgesic combination
Ilosone	Antibiotic
Ilotycin	Antibiotic
Imavate	Antidepressant (Tricyclic)
IMIPRAMINE	Antidepressant (Tricyclic)
Imodium	Antidiarrheal
Inderal	Beta Blocker
Inderide	Antihypertensive
Indocin	Nonsteroid Anti-inflammatory
INDOMETHACIN	Nonsteroid Anti-inflammatory
INSULIN	Insulin
Ionamin	Nonamphetamine Appetite Suppressant
Ismelin	Antihypertensive
Iso-Bid	Antianginal

drug	***usage***
Isobutal	Nonnarcotic analgesic combination
Isoclor Timesule	Antihistamine
Isogard	Antianginal
Isollyl	Nonnarcotic analgesic combination
Isoptin	Calcium-ion Antagonist (Antianginal)
Isordil	Antianginal
ISOSORBIDE DINITRATE	Antianginal
Isotrate	Antianginal
ISOXSUPRINE HCl	Vasodilator
Janimine	Antidepressant (Tricyclic)
Jen-Diril	Diuretic
K-Tab	Potassium Supplement
Kaon-Cl	Potassium Supplement
Kavrin	Vasodilator
Keflex	Antibiotic
Klavikordal	Antianginal

drug	usage
Klotrix	Potassium Supplement
Kolantyl	Aluminum/ Magnesium Antacid
Krem	Calcium/ Magnesium Antacid
Kudrox	Aluminum/ Magnesium Antacid
LaBID	Xanthine Bronchodilator
Lanophyllin	Xanthine Bronchodilator
Lanorinal	Nonnarcotic analgesic combination
Lanoxin	Cardiac Glycoside (Digitalis)
Lapav	Vasodilator
Lardet	Antihistamine
Larotid	Penicillin Type Antibiotic
Lasix	Potent Diuretic
Lavodopa	Anti-Parkinsonian
Leder-BP	Antihistamine/ Decongestant

drug	*usage*
Ledercillin VK	Antibiotic (Penicillin)
Lente Iletin	Insulin
LEVODOPA	Anti-Parkinsonian
Levoid	Thyroid
Levothroid	Thyroid
LEVOTHYROXINE	Thyroid
Lexor	Diuretic
Librax	Gastrointestinal Anticholinergic
Libritabs	Tranquilizer
Librium	Tranquilizer
LIMBITROL	Antidepressant (Tricyclic)
Limit	Nonamphetamine Appetite Suppressant
Liquiprin	Acetaminophen Analgesic
Liquix-C	Acetaminophen/ Narcotic Analgesic
Liquophylline	Xanthine Bronchodilator
Lithane	Antipsychotic
LITHIUM	Antipsychotic
Lithobid	Antipsychotic

drug	*usage*
Lo-Trol	Antidiarrheal
Lo/Ovral	Contraceptive
Lobac	Skeletal Muscle Relaxant
Loestrin	Contraceptive
Lofene	Antidiarrheal
Loflo	Antidiarrheal
Lomanate	Antidiarrheal
Lomotil	Antidiarrheal
Lomoxate	Antidiarrheal
Loniten	Antihypertensive
Lonox	Antidiarrheal
LOPERAMIDE	Antidiarrheal
Lopressor	Beta Blocker (Antihypertensive)
Lopurin	Antigout
LORAZEPAM	Tranquilizer
Low-Quel	Antidiarrheal
Ludiomil	Antidepressant (Tricyclic)
Luminal	Hypnotic/Sedative/ Anticonvulsant
LV Penicillin	Antibiotic (Penicillin)

drug	*usage*
M-Cillin B-400	Antibiotic (Penicillin)
M-Tetra	Antibiotic
Maalox	Aluminum/ Magnesium Antacid
Maalox Plus	Aluminum/ Magnesium/ Simethicone Antacid
Macalbis	Calcium Antacid
Macrodantin	Urinary Antibiotic
Mag-Ox 400	Magnesium Antacid
Magmalin	Aluminum/ Magnesium Antacid
Magnagel	Aluminum/ Magnesium Antacid
Magnalum	Aluminum/ Magnesium Antacid
Magnatril	Aluminum/ Magnesium Antacid
Magnesium Carbonate	Magnesium Antacid

drug	*usage*
Magnesium Oxide	Magnesium Antacid
Magnesium Trisilicate	Magnesium Antacid
Mallamint	Calcium Antacid
Maolate	Skeletal Muscle Relaxant
Maox	Magnesium Antacid
MAPROTILINE	Antidepressant (Tricyclic)
Marax	Antiasthmatic
Marbaxin	Skeletal Muscle Relaxant
Margesic Compound 65	Synthetic Narcotic Analgesic
Marnal	Nonnarcotic analgesic combination
Maxamag	Aluminum/ Magnesium Antacid
MECLIZINE	Antiemetic/ Antivertigo
Medrol	Steroid
MEDROXYPROGESTERONE	Female Hormone

drug	*usage*
Melfiat	Nonamphetamine Appetite Suppressant
Mellaril	Phenothiazine Antipsychotic
MEPERIDINE	Narcotic
MEPROBAMATE	Tranquilizer
Meprospan	Tranquilizer
Mequin	Sedative/Hypnotic
MESORIDAZINE	Phenothiazine Antipsychotic
Metandren Tablets	Male Hormone
Metaprel	Bronchodilator
METAPROTERANOL	Bronchodilator
METHAQUALONE HCl	Sedative/Hypnotic
METHENAMINE HIPPURATE	Urinary Antibiotic
Metho	Skeletal Muscle Relaxant
METHOCARBAMOL	Skeletal Muscle Relaxant
Methoxal	Urinary Antibiotic
Methoxanol	Urinary Antibiotic
METHYLCLOTHIAZIDE	Diuretic

drug	*usage*
METHYLDOPA	Antihypertensive
METHYLPHENIDATE	Central Nervous System Stimulant
METHYLPREDISOLONE	Steroid
METHYLTESTOSTERONE	Male Hormone
METHYPRYLON	Sedative/Hypnotic
Meticorten	Steroid
METOCLOPRAMIDE	Gastrointestinal Stimulant
METOPROLOL	Beta Blocker (Antihypertensive)
Metra	Nonamphetamine Appetite Suppressant
METRONIDAZOLE	Amoebicide (Trichomonas Infections)
Microsul	Urinary Antibiotic
Midatane	Antihistamine
Midatap	Antihistamine/ Decongestant
Midrin	Aspirin
Milk of Magnesia	Magnesium Antacid
Miltown	Tranquilizer
Minipress	Antihypertensive

drug	*usage*
Minocin	Antibiotic
MINOCYCLINE	Antibiotic
MINOXIDIL	Antihypertensive
Mint-o-Mag	Magnesium Antacid
Modicon	Contraceptive
Moduretic	Diuretic (Antihypertensive)
Monacet with Codeine	Narcotic Analgesic/Cough Suppressant
Motion Cure	Antiemetic/ Antivertigo
Motrin	Nonsteroid Anti-inflammatory
Murcil	Tranquilizer
Mylanta	Aluminum/ Magnesium/ Simethicone Antacid
Myobid	Vasodilator
Mysoline	Anticonvulsant
NADOLOL	Beta Blocker
Naldecon Tablets	Antihistamine/ Decongestant
Nalfon	Anti-inflammatory

drug	*usage*
Naprosyn	Nonsteroid Anti-inflammatory
NAPROXEN	Nonsteroid Anti-inflammatory
Navane	Antipsychotic
Nembutal	Hypnotic/Sedative
NeoFed	Bronchodilator/ Decongestant
Neopap Supprettes	Acetaminophen Analgesic
Nephrox	Aluminum Antacid
Neuramate	Tranquilizer
Neutracomp	Aluminum/ Magnesium Antacid
Neutralox	Aluminum/ Magnesium Antacid
NIFEDIPINE	Calcium-ion Antagonist (Antianginal)
Niong	Antianginal
Nitrex	Urinary Antibiotic
Nitro-Bid	Antianginal
Nitro-Dur Patches	Antianginal
Nitro-T.D.	Antianginal

drug	*usage*
Nitrocap T.D.	Antianginal
Nitrodan	Urinary Antibiotic
Nitrodisc	Antianginal
NITROFURANTOIN	Urinary Antibiotic
NITROGLYCERIN	Antianginal
Nitrol	Antianginal
Nitrolin	Antianginal
Nitronet	Antianginal
Nitrong	Antianginal
Nitrospan	Antianginal
Nitrostat	Antianginal
Noctec	Sedative/Hypnotic
Noludar	Sedative/Hypnotic
Nor-Mil	Antidiarrheal
Nor-Tet	Antibiotic
Nordryl	Antihistamine
Norgesic	Muscle Relaxant Combination
Norinyl	Contraceptive
Norlestrin	Contraceptive
Normatane	Antihistamine/ Decongestant

drug	*usage*
Norpanth	Gastrointestinal Anticholinergic Agent
Norpramin	Antidepressant (Tricyclic)
NORTRIPTYLINE	Antidepressant (Tricyclic)
NOSCAPINE	Cough Suppressant
Novafed	Bronchodilator/ Decongestant
Novahistine LP	Antihistamine/ Decongestant
NPH Iletin	Insulin
Obalan	Nonamphetamine Appetite Suppressant
Obepal	Nonamphetamine Appetite Suppressant
Obepar	Nonamphetamine Appetite Suppressant
Obephen	Nonamphetamine Appetite Suppressant
Obetrol	Nonamphetamine Appetite Suppressant

drug	*usage*
Obezine	Nonamphetamine Appetite Suppressant
Omnibese	Nonamphetamine Appetite Suppressant
Omnipen	Penicillin Type Antibiotic
Optimine	Antihistamine
Ora-Testryl	Male Hormone
Oradrate	Sedative/Hypnotic
Oralphyllin	Xanthine Bronchodilator
Orapav Timecelles	Vasodilator
Oraphen-PD	Acetaminophen Analgesic
Orasone	Steroid
Oretic	Diuretic
Oreton	Male Hormone
Orinase	Antidiabetic
Ormazine	Phenothiazine Tranquilizer
Ornade	Antihistamine/ Decongestant
Ortho-Novum	Contraceptive
Os-Cal	Mineral Supplement

drug	*usage*
Ovcon	Contraceptive
Ovral	Contraceptive
Ovulen	Contraceptive
Oxabid	Magnesium Antacid
OXACILLIN SODIUM	Antibiotic
Oxalid	Anti-inflammatory
OXAZEPAM	Tranquilizer
OXTRIPHYLLINE	Xanthine Bronchodilator
OXYMETAZOLINE HCl	Nasal Decongestant
OXYPHENBUTAZONE	Anti-inflammatory
P.H. Tablets	Calcium Antacid
P-A-C Compound	Narcotic Analgesic/Cough Suppressant
Paltet	Antibiotic
PAMA	Aluminum/ Magnesium Antacid
Pamelor	Antidepressant (Tricyclic)
Panahist	Antihistamine
Panasol	Steroid

drug	*usage*
Panelex	Acetaminophen/ Narcotic Analgesic
Panex	Acetaminophen Analgesic
Panmycin	Antibiotic
Panwarfin	Anticoagulant
Papa-Deine	Acetaminophen/ Narcotic Analgesic
Papa-Deine Tablets	Narcotic Analgesic/Cough Suppressant
PAPAVERINE	Vasodilator
Par-Mag	Magnesium Antacid
Parachlor	Skeletal Muscle Relaxant
Parafon Forte	Skeletal Muscle Relaxant
PAREGORIC	Narcotic Antidiarrheal
Parest	Sedative/Hypnotic
Pargesic 65	Synthetic Narcotic
Parmine	Nonamphetamine Appetite Suppressant
Partrex	Antibiotic

drug	usage
Pathocil	Antibiotic
Pava-Mead	Vasodilator
Pava-RX	Vasodilator
Pavabid	Vasodilator
Pavacap Unicelles	Vasodilator
Pavacen Cenules	Vasodilator
Pavadon Elixir	Acetaminophen/ Narcotic Analgesic
Pavadur	Vasodilator
Pavadyl	Vasodilator
Pavagen	Vasodilator
Pavakey	Vasodilator
Pavased	Vasodilator
Pavasule	Vasodilator
Pavatym	Vasodilator
Paverine-Spancaps	Vasodilator
Paverolan	Vasodilator
Paxipam	Tranquilizer
PBR/12	Hypnotic/Sedative/ Anticonvulsant
PBZ	Antihistamine
PDM	Nonamphetamine Appetite Suppressant

drug	*usage*
PE-DE-EM	Nonamphetamine Appetite Suppressant
Pediamycin	Antibiotic
Pedric Wafers	Acetaminophen Analgesic
PEMOLINE	Psychotherapeutic
Pen-Vee K	Antibiotic (Penicillin)
Penapar VK	Antibiotic (Penicillin)
Penbritin	Penicillin Type Antibiotic
PENICILLIN G	Antibiotic (Penicillin)
Pensyn	Penicillin Type Antibiotic
PENTAZOCINE	Synthetic Analgesic
Pentids	Antibiotic (Penicillin)
PENTOBARBITAL	Hypnotic/Sedative
Percocet	Narcotic Analgesic Combination
Percodan	Narcotic Analgesic Combination
Peri-Colace	Laxative

drug	*usage*
Periactin	Phenothiazine-type Antihistamine
Permitil	Phenothiazine Antipsychotic
Persantine	Antianginal
Pertofrane	Antidepressant (Tricyclic)
Pfizer-E	Antibiotic
Pfizerpen A	Penicillin Type Antibiotic
Pfizerpen G	Antibiotic (Penicillin)
Pfizerpen VK	Antibiotic (Penicillin)
Phedral	Antihistamine
Phen-Azo	Urinary Analgesic
Phenaphen	Acetaminophen Analgesic
Phenazine	Nonamphetamine Appetite Suppressant
Phenazodine	Urinary Analgesic
PHENAZOPYRIDINE HCl	Urinary Analgesic
Phendimead	Nonamphetamine Appetite Suppressant

drug	*usage*
PHENDIMETRAZINE	Nonamphetamine Appetite Suppressant
PhenaPhen with Codeine	Acetaminophen/ Narcotic Analgesic
Phenetron	Antihistamine
Pheno-Squar	Hypnotic/Sedative/ Anticonvulsant
PHENOBARBITAL	Hypnotic/Sedative/ Anticonvulsant
PHENTERMINE HCl	Nonamphetamine Appetite Suppressant
Phentrol	Nonamphetamine Appetite Suppressant
PHENYLBUTAZONE	Anti-inflammatory
PHENYTOIN	Anticonvulsant
Phenzine	Nonamphetamine Appetite Suppressant
Phosphaljel	Aluminum Antacid
Physpan	Xanthine Bronchodilator
PIROXICAM	Non-steroid Anti-inflammatory
Placidyl	Sedative/Hypnotic

drug	*usage*
Polaramine	Antihistamine
Polycillin	Penicillin Type Antibiotic
Polymox	Penicillin Type Antibiotic
POTASSIUM CHLORIDE	Potassium Supplement
Potassium CL	Potassium Supplement
PRAZEPAM	Tranquilizer
PRAZOSIN	Antihypertensive
Prednicen-M	Steroid
PREDNISONE	Steroid
Prelu-2	Nonamphetamine Appetite Suppressant
Premarin	Female Hormone
Presamine	Antidepressant (Tricyclic)
Primatene "P"	Antihistamine
PRIMIDONE	Anticonvulsant
Principen	Penicillin Type Antibiotic
Pro-Banthine	Gastrointestinal Anticholinergic Agent
PROCAINAMIDE HCl	Antiarrhythmic

drug	*usage*
Procan	Antiarrhythmic
Procardia	Calcium-ion Antagonist (Antianginal)
PROCHLORPERAZINE	Phenothiazine Anti-Emetic/ Antipsychotic
Progesic Compound-65	Synthetic Narcotic Analgesic
Proklar	Urinary Antibiotic
Prolixin	Phenothiazine Antipsychotic
Proloid	Thyroid Replacement
Promapar	Phenothiazine Tranquilizer
Promaz	Phenothiazine Tranquilizer
Pronestyl	Antiarrhythmic
PROPANTHELINE	Gastrointestinal Anticholinergic Agent
PROPOXYPHENE HCl	Synthetic Narcotic
PROPRANOLOL HCl	Beta Blocker
Prostaphlin	Antibiotic
Protran	Tranquilizer
PROTRIPTYLINE HCl	Antidepressant (Tricyclic)

drug	***usage***
Proval	Acetaminophen/ Narcotic Analgesic
Provera	Female Hormone
Proxagesic	Synthetic Narcotic
Proxagesic Compound-65	Synthetic Narcotic Analgesic
Proxene	Synthetic Narcotic
Pruodigin	Cardiac Glycoside (Digitalis)
PSEUDOEPHEDRINE	Bronchodilator/ Decongestant
Psychozine	Phenothiazine Tranquilizer
Puretane	Antihistamine
Puretapp	Antihistamine/ Decongestant
Pyribenzamine	Antihistamine
Pyridiate	Urinary Analgesic
Pyridium	Urinary Analgesic
Pyrodine	Urinary Analgesic
Quaalude	Sedative/Hypnotic
Quibron	Antihistamine
Quinidex	Antiarrhythmic
QUINIDINE SULFATE	Antiarrhythmic
Quinora	Antiarrhythmic

drug	*usage*
R-HCTZ-H	Antihypertensive
Ratio	Calcium/ Magnesium Antacid
Reglan	Gastrointestinal Stimulant
Regroton	Antihypertensive
Rela	Skeletal Muscle Relaxant
Repen-VK	Antibiotic (Penicillin)
Respirol	Antihistamine
Restoril	Sedative/Sleeping Agent
Retet	Antibiotic
Retin-A	Antiacne
Reton	Nonamphetamine Appetite Suppressant
Rifadin	Anti-Tuberculosis
RIFAMPIN	Anti-Tuberculosis
Rimactane	Anti-Tuberculosis
Riopan	Aluminum/ Magnesium Antacid
Ritalin	Central Nervous System Stimulant

drug	*usage*
RITODRINE	Uterine Relaxant
Robalate	Aluminum Antacid
Robamol	Skeletal Muscle Relaxant
Robamox	Penicillin Type Antibiotic
Robaxin	Skeletal Muscle Relaxant
Robicillin VK	Antibiotic (Penicillin)
Robimycin	Antibiotic
Robitet	Antibiotic
Rolaids	Aluminum Antacid
Rolox	Aluminum/ Magnesium Antacid
Ropanth	Gastrointestinal Anticholinergic Agent
RP-Mycin	Antibiotic
Rulox	Aluminum/ Magnesium Antacid
S.A.S.-500	Sulfonamide
Salatin with Codeine	Narcotic Analgesic/Cough Suppressant

drug	*usage*
Salutensin	Antihypertensive
Sarisol	Hypnotic/Sedative/ Anticonvulsant
Scrip-Dyne Compound	Synthetic Narcotic Analgesic
SECOBARBITAL	Hypnotic/Sedative
Seconal	Hypnotic/Sedative
Sedabamate	Tranquilizer
Sedadrops	Hypnotic/Sedative/ Anticonvulsant
Septra	Urinary Antibiotic
Sequels	Antihistamine/ Decongestant
Ser Hydra Zine	Antihypertensive
Ser-A-Gen	Antihypertensive
Ser-Ap-Es	Antihypertensive
Seralazide	Antihypertensive
Serax	Tranquilizer
Sereen	Tranquilizer
Serentil	Phenothiazine Antipsychotic
Silain Gel	Aluminum/ Magnesium/ Simethicone Antacid

drug	usage
Simaal	Aluminum/ Magnesium/ Simethicone Antacid
Simeco	Aluminum/ Magnesium/ Simethicone Antacid
Sinemet	Anti-Parkinsonian
Sinequan	Antidepressant (Tricyclic)
Singlet Tablets	Decongestant/ Antihistamine
Sinubid	Decongestant/ Antihistamine
Sinufed	Bronchodilator/ Decongestant
SK Amitriptyline	Antidepressant (Tricyclic)
SK-Ampicillin	Penicillin Type Antibiotic
SK-APAP	Acetaminophen Analgesic
SK-APAP with Codeine	Acetaminophen/ Narcotic Analgesic
SK-Chlorothiazide	Diuretic
SK-Lygen	Tranquilizer
SK-65 Compound	Synthetic Narcotic Analgesic

drug	*usage*
SK-65 Capsules	Synthetic Narcotic
Slo-Phyllin	Xanthine Bronchodilator
Slow-K	Potassium Supplement
Soda Mint	Sodium Bicarbonate Antacid
Sodestrin-H	Female Hormone
Sodium Amytal	Hypnotic/Sedative/ Anticonvulsant
Sodium Bicarbonate	Sodium Bicarbonate Antacid
Soduben	Hypnotic/Sedative/ Anticonvulsant
Solfoton	Hypnotic/Sedative/ Anticonvulsant
Soma	Skeletal Muscle Relaxant
Somophyllin	Xanthine Bronchodilator
Sorate	Antianginal
Sorbide T.D.	Antianginal
Sorbitrate	Antianginal
Spancap	Amphetamine

drug	*usage*
Spastosed	Calcium/ Magnesium Antacid
Spenaxin	Skeletal Muscle Relaxant
Spengine	Psychotherapeutic for Elderly
Spenox	Aluminum/ Magnesium Antacid
Spentane	Antihistamine
Sperx	Nonamphetamine Appetite Suppressant
Spiractazide	Diuretic
Spiractone	Diuretic
Spironazide	Diuretic
SPIRONOLACTONE	Diuretic
Statobex	Nonamphetamine Appetite Suppressant
Stelazine	Phenothiazine Antipsychotic
Sterapred	Steroid
Stilbestrol	Female Hormone (Estrogen)

drug	*usage*
Stim-35	Nonamphetamine Appetite Suppressant
Sub-Quin	Antiarrhythmic
SUCRALFATE	Anti-Ulcer
Sudafed	Bronchodilator/ Decongestant
Sudoprin	Acetaminophen Analgesic
Sudrin	Bronchodilator/ Decongestant
Suhist Tablets	Antihistamine/ Decongestant
Suldiazo	Urinary Antibiotic
Sulfadyne	Sulfonamide
SULFAMETHIZOLE	Urinary Antibiotic
SULFAMETHOXAZOLE	Urinary Antibiotic
SULFASALAZINE	Sulfonamide
Sulfasox	Urinary Antibiotic
SULFISOXAZOLE	Urinary Antibiotic
Sulfizin	Urinary Antibiotic
SULINDAC	Nonsteroid Anti-inflammatory
Sumox	Penicillin Type Antibiotic

drug	*usage*
Sumycin	Antibiotic
Supen	Penicillin Type Antibiotic
Surmontil	Antidepressant (Tricyclic)
Suspen	Antibiotic (Penicillin)
Sustaire	Xanthine Bronchodilator
Symptom 2	Bronchodilator/Deconges[illegible]
Symptom 3	Antihistamine
Synalgos-DC	Narcotic Analgesic Combination
Synthroid	Thyroid
Syntrogel	Aluminum/ Magnesium Antacid
T.D. Alermine	Antihistamine
T.E.P. Tablets	Antihistamine
T.H.P. Tablets	Anticholinergic
T-E-P Compound	Antihistamine
T-250	Antibiotic
Tabloid APC	Narcotic Analgesic/Cough Suppressant

drug	*usage*
Tagatap	Antihistamine/ Decongestant
Tagamet	Anti-Ulcer (H2 Antagonist)
Talwin	Synthetic Analgesic
Tandearil	Anti-inflammatory
Tapar	Acetaminophen Analgesic
Tedral	Antihistamine
Teldrin Spansules	Antihistamine
TEMAZEPAM	Sedative/Sleeping Agent
Tempra	Acetaminophen Analgesic
Ten-Shun	Nonnarcotic analgesic combination
Tenax	Tranquilizer
Tenol	Acetaminophen Analgesic
Tenormin	Beta Blocker
Tenuate	Nonamphetamine Appetite Suppressant
Tepanil	Nonamphetamine Appetite Suppressant

drug	*usage*
TERBUTALINE SULFATE	Bronchodilator
TERPIN HYDRATE	Cough Suppressant
Terrastatin	Antibiotic
Testred	Male Hormone
Tet-250	Antibiotic
Tetra-Bid	Antibiotic
Tetra-C	Antibiotic
Tetra-Co	Antibiotic
Tetracap	Antibiotic
Tetrachel	Antibiotic
TETRACYCLINE	Antibiotic
Tetracyn	Antibiotic
Tetralan-250	Antibiotic
Tetram	Antibiotic
Tetrex bidCAPS	Antibiotic
Theo-dur	Xanthine Bronchodilator
Theobid	Xanthine Bronchodilator
Theocap	Xanthine Bronchodilator
Theoclear	Xanthine Bronchodilator
Theodrine	Antihistamine

drug	usage
Theofedral	Antihistamine
Theofenal	Antihistamine
Theolair	Xanthine Bronchodilator
Theolixir	Xanthine Bronchodilator
Theon	Xanthine Bronchodilator
Theophenyllin	Antihistamine
Theophyl	Xanthine Bronchodilator
THEOPHYLLINE	Xanthine Bronchodilator
Theoral	Antihistamine
Theospan	Xanthine Bronchodilator
Theostat	Xanthine Bronchodilator
Theovent	Xanthine Bronchodilator
Therapan	Vasodilator
Thermoloid	Thyroid Replacement
THIOGUANINE	Anti-Leukemia
THIORIDAZINE HCl	Phenothiazine Antipsychotic
Thiosulful	Urinary Antibiotic

drug	*usage*
THIOTHIXENE	Antipsychotic
Thorazine	Phenothiazine Tranquilizer
Thyrocrine	Thyroid Replacement
THYROGLOBULIN	Thyroid Replacement
THYROID	Thyroid Replacement
Thyrolar	Thyroid
Tigan	Antiemetic
TIMOLOL	Beta Blocker
Titralac	Calcium Antacid
Tofranil	Antidepressant (Tricyclic)
TOLAZAMIDE	Antidiabetic
TOLBUTAMIDE	Antidiabetic
Tolectin	Nonsteroid Anti-inflammatory
Tolinase	Antidiabetic
TOLMETIN	Nonsteroid Anti-inflammatory
Tora	Nonamphetamine Appetite Suppressant
Totacillin	Penicillin Type Antibiotic

drug	*usage*
Tralmag	Aluminum/ Magnesium Antacid
Tranmep	Tranquilizer
Transderm Nitro	Antianginal
Tranxene	Tranquilizer
Trates Granucaps	Antianginal
Tremin	Anticholinergic
TRETINOIN	Antiacne
Trihexane	Anticholinergic
Tri-Hydroserpine	Antihypertensive
Tri-Pavasule	Vasodilator
Trialka Liquid	Aluminum/ Magnesium Antacid
Trialka Tablets	Calcium Antacid
Triavil	Antidepressant (Tricyclic)
TRIFLUOPERAZINE	Phenothiazine Antipsychotic
Trihexidyl	Anticholinergic
TRIHEXYPHENIDYL HCl	Anticholinergic
Trimagel	Aluminum/ Magnesium Antacid
TRIMETHOBENZAMIDE	Antiemetic

drug	*usage*
TRIMETHOPRIM	Urinary Antibiotic
TRIMIPRAMINE	Antidepressant (Tricyclic)
Trimox	Penicillin Type Antibiotic
Trimpex	Urinary Antibiotic
Trimstat	Nonamphetamine Appetite Suppressant
Trimtabs	Nonamphetamine Appetite Suppressant
TRIPELENNAMINE	Antihistamine
Trisogel	Aluminum/ Magnesium Antacid
Trymegen	Antihistamine
Tuinal	Hypnotic
Tuloidin	Thyroid Replacement
Tumol	Skeletal Muscle Relaxant
Tums	Calcium Antacid
Tuss-Ornade	Decongestant/ Expectorant
Tusscapine	Cough Suppressant

drug	usage
Tuzon	Skeletal Muscle Relaxant
Twinbarbital	Hypnotic
Tylenol	Acetaminophen Analgesic
Tylenol with Codeine	Acetaminophen/Narcotic Analgesic
Tylox	Narcotic Analgesic Combination
Unifast Unicelles	Nonamphetamine Appetite Suppressant
Unipres	Antihypertensive
Uro-Mag	Magnesium Antacid
Urex	Urinary Antibiotic
Urifon	Urinary Antibiotic
Urotoin	Urinary Antibiotic
Uticillin VK	Antibiotic (Penicillin)
V-Cillin K	Antibiotic (Penicillin)
Valadol	Acetaminophen Analgesic
Valdrene	Antihistamine
Valium	Tranquilizer

drug	usage
Valorin	Acetaminophen Analgesic
VALPROIC ACID	Anticonvulsant
Vanceril	Steroid
Vasal Granucaps	Vasodilator
Vasocap	Vasodilator
Vasodilan	Vasodilator
Vasoprine	Vasodilator
Vasospan	Vasodilator
Veetids	Antibiotic (Penicillin)
Velosef	Antibiotic
Veltane	Antihistamine
Veracillin	Antibiotic
VERAPAMIL	Calcium-ion Antagonist (Antianginal)
Vibramycin	Antibiotic
Virilon	Male Hormone
Vistaril	Antihistamine/ Antinausea/ Antianxiety
Vivactil	Antidepressant (Tricyclic)
WARFARIN	Anticoagulant

drug	*usage*
Weh-less	Nonamphetamine Appetite Suppressant
Wehvert	Antiemetic/ Antivertigo
Weightrol	Nonamphetamine Appetite Suppressant
Wilpowr	Nonamphetamine Appetite Suppressant
WinGel	Aluminum/ Magnesium Antacid
Wyamycin	Antibiotic
Wygesic	Synthetic Narcotic
Wymox	Penicillin Type Antibiotic
Xanax	Tranquilizer
Yutopar	Uterine Relaxant
Zetran	Tranquilizer
Zide	Diuretic
Zomax	Nonnarcotic Synthetic Analgesic
ZOMEPIRAC	Nonnarcotic Synthetic Analgesic

drug	***usage***
Zovirax	Antiviral
Zyloprim	Antigout

6

EMERGENCY TREATMENT PROTOCOLS

The algorithms on the following pages are adapted from the Instructors' Manual for Advanced Cardiac Life Support, American Heart Association, Dallas, Texas, pp 441-453, 1982

Figure 6-1. Cardiac Arrest—Adults

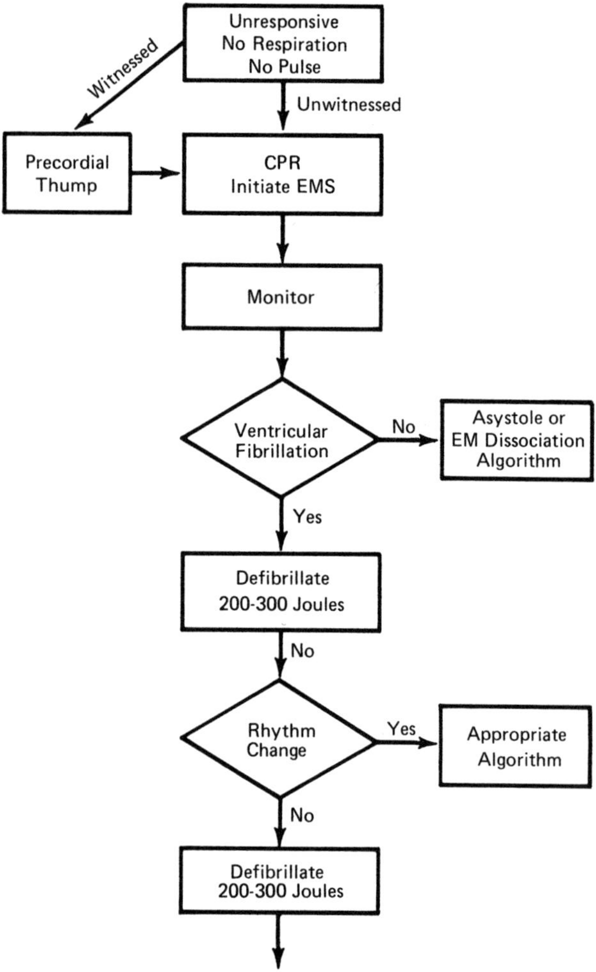

(Continued)

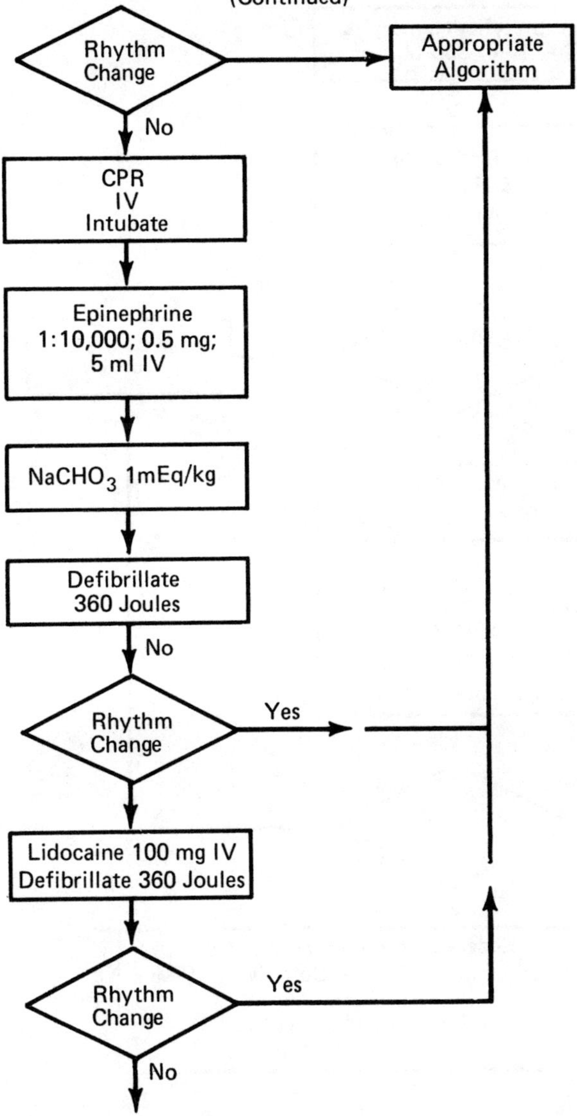
Rhythm Change
Appropriate Algorithm
No
CPR
IV
Intubate
Epinephrine
1:10,000; 0.5 mg;
5 ml IV
NaCHO3 1mEq/kg
Defibrillate
360 Joules
No
Rhythm Change
Yes
Lidocaine 100 mg IV
Defibrillate 360 Joules
Rhythm Change
Yes
No

(Continued)

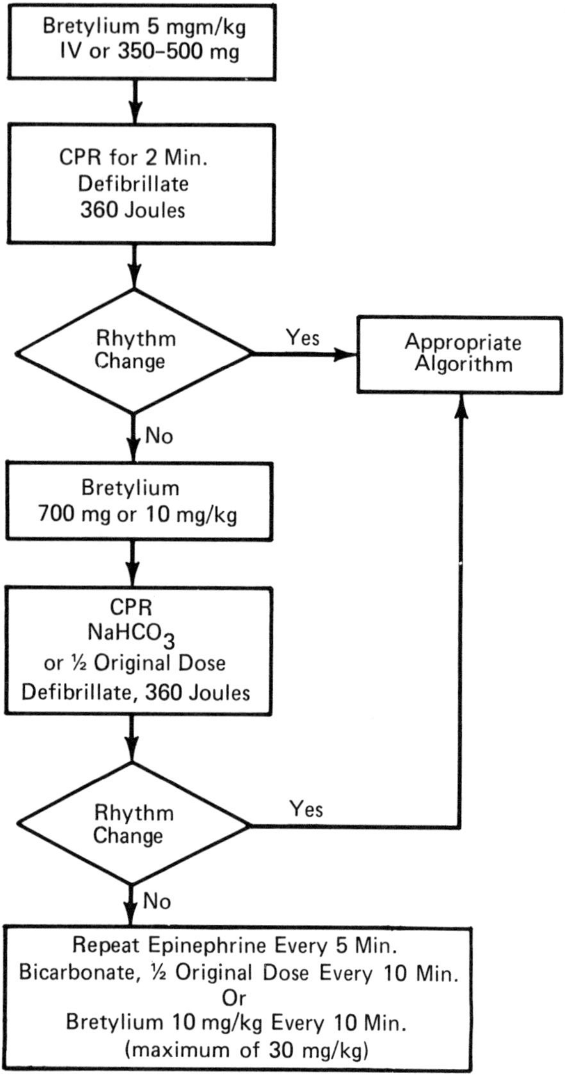
Bretylium 5 mgm/kg IV or 350–500 mg
CPR for 2 Min. Defibrillate 360 Joules
Rhythm Change
Yes
Appropriate Algorithm
No
Bretylium 700 mg or 10 mg/kg
CPR $NaHCO_3$ or ½ Original Dose Defibrillate, 360 Joules
Rhythm Change
Yes
No
Repeat Epinephrine Every 5 Min. Bicarbonate, ½ Original Dose Every 10 Min. Or Bretylium 10 mg/kg Every 10 Min. (maximum of 30 mg/kg)

Figure 6-2. Ventricular Tachycardia

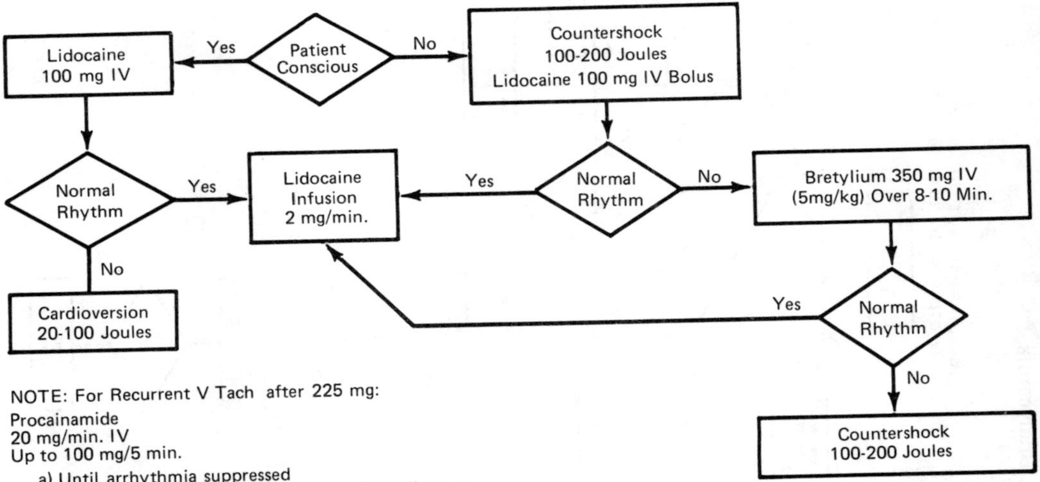

NOTE: For Recurrent V Tach after 225 mg:

Procainamide
20 mg/min. IV
Up to 100 mg/5 min.

a) Until arrhythmia suppressed
b) Or hypotension ensues
c) Or QRS widens by 50%
d) Or a total of 1 gm

Follow With Infusion
Of procainamide 1-4 mg/min

or

Bretylium
5 mg/kg IV Bolus

Figure 6-3. Bradycardia

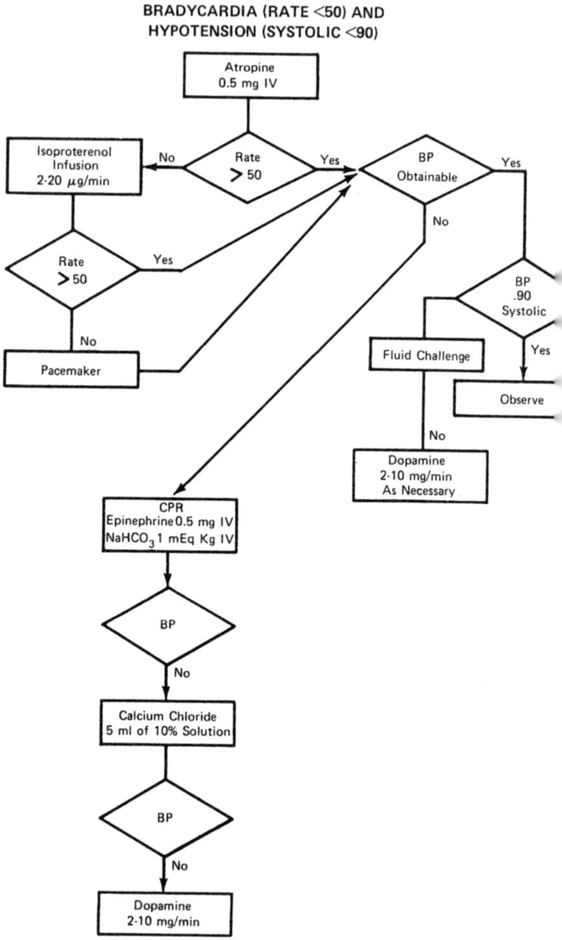

Figure 6-4. Asystole

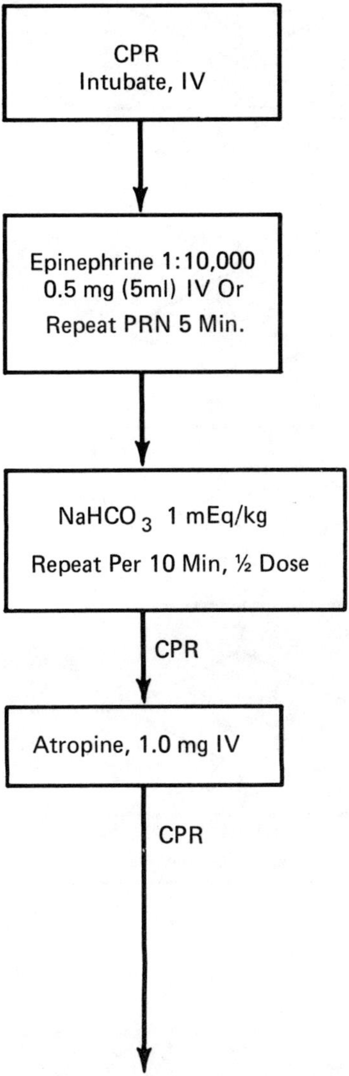

(Continued)

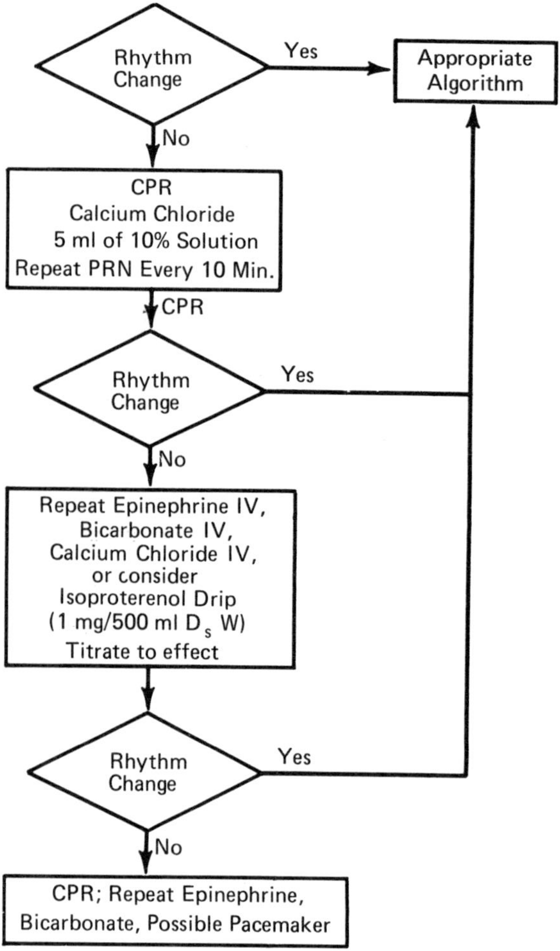
Rhythm Change
Yes
Appropriate Algorithm
No
CPR
Calcium Chloride
5 ml of 10% Solution
Repeat PRN Every 10 Min.
CPR
Rhythm Change
Yes
No
Repeat Epinephrine IV,
Bicarbonate IV,
Calcium Chloride IV,
or consider
Isoproterenol Drip
(1 mg/500 ml D5 W)
Titrate to effect
Rhythm Change
Yes
No
CPR; Repeat Epinephrine,
Bicarbonate, Possible Pacemaker

Figure 6-5. Electromechanical Dissociation

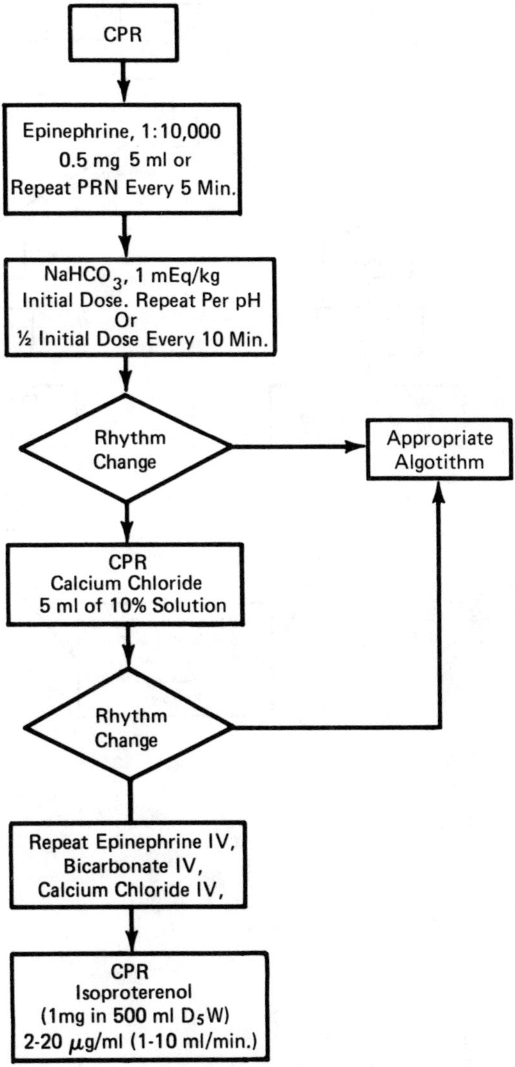

Figure 6-6. Malignant Premature Ventricular Contractions

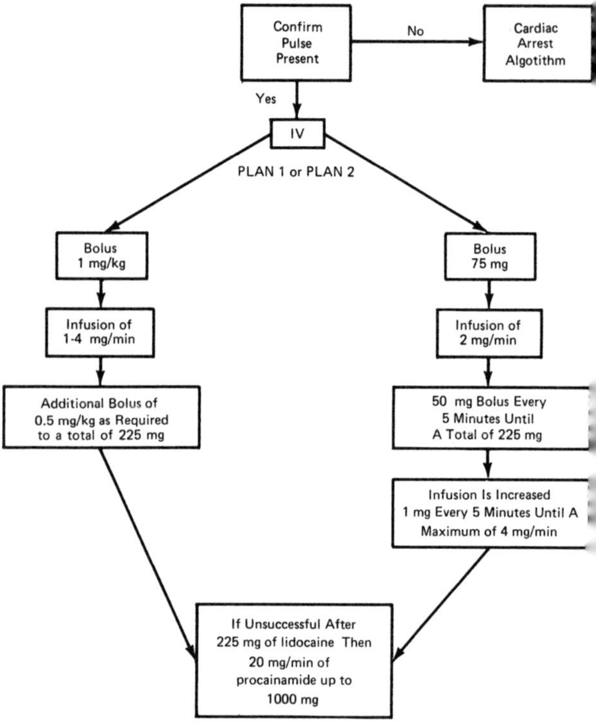

REFERENCES

REFERENCES

AMA Department of Drugs: AMA Drug Evaluation, 4th ed. Publishing Sciences Group, Inc., Littleton, Massachusetts, 1980

American Heart Association: Textbook of Advanced Cardiac Life Support, 2nd ed. American Heart Association, Dallas, Texas, 1981

American Pharmaceutical Association, National Formulary Board: National Formulary, 15th ed. W.B. Saunders Co., Philadelphia, Pennsylvania, 1980

Asperheim M, Eisenhauer L: The Pharmacological Basis of Patient Care, 3rd ed. W.B. Saunders Co., Philadelphia, Pennsylvania, 1977

Bruce C, Gutierrez-Mazorra J: Pediatric Emergency Drug Manual CPR. The Childrens Hospital of Alabama, Birmingham, Alabama

Goodman L, Gilman A: The Pharmacological Basis of Therapeutics, 6th ed. The MacMillan Publishing Co., New York, New York, 1980

Goth A: Medical Pharmacology; Principles and Concepts, 9th ed. The C.V. Mosby Co., St. Louis, Missouri, 1978

Guyton A: Textbook of Medical Physiology, 6th ed. The W.B. Saunders Co., Philadelphia, Pennsylvania, 1981

Huzar R: Emergency Cardiac Care, 2nd ed. Robert J. Brady Co., Bowie, Maryland, 1982

Physicians Desk Reference, 36th ed. Medical Economics Co., Oradell, New Jersey, 1982

Safar P: Cardiopulmonary Cerebral Resuscitation The W.B. Saunders Co., Philadelphia, Pennsylvania, 1981

Texas College of Osteopathic Medicine, Department of Pharmacology: A Guide to Experimental Pharmacology. Fort Worth, Texas 1980

United States Pharmacopeial Convention: United States Pharmacopia, 20th ed. Washington, D.C., 1980

Walraven G et al: Manual of Advanced Prehospital Care. Robert J. Brady Co., Bowie, Maryland, 1978

APPENDICES

PHARMACOLOGICAL ABBREVIATIONS

It is common to use abbreviations in pharmacology. This serves to expedite paper work and promote efficiency. The abbreviations used in pharmacology are fairly standard. It is important to be familiar with these abbreviations and with some of the common terminology applicable to the field of emergency pharmacology.

abbreviation	***meaning***
$\bar{a}$	before
ACh	acetylcholine
ACLS	advanced cardiac life support
ALS	advanced life support
amp	ampule
α	alpha
ASA	aspirin
b.i.d.	two times a day
BLS	basic life support
β	beta
$\bar{c}$	with
c/o	complains of
Ca^{++}	calcium ion
$CaCl_2$	calcium chloride
caps	capsules
cc	cubic centimeter
CHF	congestive heart failure
Cl^-	chlorine ion
cm	centimeter
cm^3	cubic centimeter
CO	carbon monoxide
COPD	chronic obstructive pulmonary disease

abbreviation	*meaning*
CSM	carotid sinus massage
CVA	cerebrovascular accident
CO_2	carbon dioxide
D/C	discontinue
dig	digitalis
DO	doctor of osteopathic medicine
Dx	diagnosis
D_5W	5% dextrose in water
$D_{50}W$	50% dextrose
EKG	electrocardiogram
elix.	elixer
EOA	esophageal obturator airway
et	and
ET	endotracheal tube
ETOH	ethyl alcohol
°F	Fahrenheit
gm	gram
gr	grain
gtts	drops
GYN	gynecological
IC	intracardiac
IM	intramuscular
IV	intravenous
K^+	potassium ion
kg	kilogram
KO	keep open
KVO	keep vein open
l	liter
lb.	pound
LBBB	left bundle branch block
LR	lactated Ringer's
MD	doctor of medicine
mEq	milliequivalents
mg	milligram
min	minute
ml	milliliter
mm	millimeter

abbreviation	*meaning*
MS	morphine sulfate
Na^+	sodium ion
$NaHCO_3$	sodium bicarbonate
nitro	nitroglycerin
NKA	no known allergies
non rep.	not to be repeated
NTG	nitroglycerin
N_20	nitrous oxide
OB	obstetric
OD	overdose
μg	microgram
μm	micrometer
OPP	organophosphate poisoning
oz.	ounce
O_2	oxygen
P	after
PAC	premature atrial contraction
PAT	paroxysmal atrial tachycardia
pedi	pediatric
PJC	premature junctional contraction
po	by mouth
pr	per rectum
prn	as needed
PSVT	paroxysmal supraventricular tachycardia
PVC	premature ventricular contraction
$\bar{q}$	every
q.h.	every hour
q.i.d.	four times a day
qt.	quart
RBBB	right bundle branch block
RL	Ringer's lactate
Rx	treatment
$\bar{s}$	without
SC	subcutaneous
Sig.	let it be labeled
SL	sublingual

abbreviation	*meaning*
sol.	solution
stat	immediately
sub q	subcutaneous
t.i.d.	three times a day
TKO	to keep open
TT	transtracheal
u.	unit
ut dict.	as directed

TRAVENOL CONVERSION TABLE

gtt/Min (10 gtt/ml)	*Rate of Infusion ml/hr*
5.0	30
	35
6.0	40
7.0	45
8.0	50
10.0	60
11.0	65
12.0	70
	75
13.0	80
15.0	90
17.0	100
20.0	120
21.0	125
23.0	140
25.0	150
33.0	200
42.0	250

(*From* Walraven G et al: Manual of Advanced Prehospital Care. Robert J. Brady Co., Bowie, Maryland, 1978)

METRIC CONVERSION TABLES

Liquid Equivalents

metric system	*apothecary system*
1000 ml (1 liter)	= 1 quart (32 fl oz)
500 ml	= 1 pint (16 fl oz)
250 ml	= 1 cup (8 fl oz)
30 ml	= 1 fluid ounce
15 ml	= 1 Tablespoon (Tbs)
4-5 ml	= 1 teaspoon (fluid dram)
1 ml = 1 cc	= 15 minims

CONVERSIONS

A. To convert cc to Tbs divide by 15 cc
Example: 45 cc ÷ 15 cc/Tbs = 3 Tbs

B. To convert Tbs to cc multiply by 15 cc
Example: 6 Tbs × 15 cc/Tbs = 90 cc

(*From* Walraven G et al: Manual of Advanced Prehospital Care. Robert J. Brady Co., Bowie, Maryland, 1978)

Weight Equivalents

metric system	*apothecary system*
1 kilogram (kg)	= 2.2 pounds (lb)
	1 pound = 16 ounces (oz)
30 gm	= 1 oz
1 gm = 1000 mg	= 15 grains
60 mg	= 1 grain
1 mg	= 1/60 grain

CONVERSIONS

A. To convert mg to grains divide by 60
Example: 300 mg ÷ 60 = 5 grains

B. To convert grains to mg multiply by 60
Example: 0.25 grains × 60 = 15 grains

C. To convert lb to kg divide by 2.2
Example: 77 lb ÷ 2.2 = 35 kg

D. To convert kg to lb multiply by 2.2
Example: 40 kg × 2.2 = 88 lb

E. To convert mg to gm divide by 1000
Example: 6000 mg ÷ 1000 = 6 gm

F. To convert gm to mg multiply by 1000
Example: 1 gm × 1000 = 1000 mg

(*From* Walraven G et al: Manual of Advanced Prehospital Care. Robert J. Brady Co., Bowie, Maryland, 1978)

INDEX

Index

A

B

C

D

E

F

G

H

I

L

M

N